Bladder Cancer
A Resource Guide for Patients and
Their Families

By

Gary N. Dunetz M.D., FACS

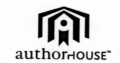

authorHOUSE™

1663 LIBERTY DRIVE, SUITE 200
BLOOMINGTON, INDIANA 47403
(800) 839-8640
WWW.AUTHORHOUSE.COM

First published by AuthorHouse 8/7/2006

ISBN: 1-4208-6365-7 (sc)

Printed in the United States of America
Bloomington, Indiana

This book is printed on acid-free paper.

To Yvonne

Thank you Danielle Dunetz D.O. for editing this book.

TABLE OF CONTENTS

CHAPTER ONE
INTRODUCTION

After the initial shock of being given a new diagnosis of cancer, a flood of emotions follow with fear and anxiety being foremost. Questions fill your mind:

How serious is it?
Can I be cured?
Am I going to die?
Will I suffer?
What treatments are available?
Can I do anything to improve my odds?
What side effects will occur from the treatments?
Will I lose time from work?
Will my insurance cover the cost?
Will I be disfigured?
Will my spouse and family be supportive?
Do I have a good doctor?

Bladder cancer, or any serious potentially life threatening illness is generally alien to most individuals. Suddenly, lives are changed and a new reality must be dealt with. Becoming a "patient" or worse "a cancer patient" is not only threatening, but a dreaded proposition. Cancer patients are not happy with the loss of autonomy, the invasion of privacy, the discomfort inflicted upon them and the demands on their time and quality of life. As a patient, being thrust into this altered identity, it is essential to seek out the information you need. Having a fundamental base of knowledge is a must when facing the issues and treatment decisions which lie ahead. In the following pages, together we will explore bladder cancer, a disease which is totally foreign to most of us until the diagnosis is made. I have chosen to present the information in a question and answer format, written in a conversational tone, as if I were having an extended consultation with one of my patients. The questions are typical of what individuals have asked over the years. I have covered the key issues and decisions the individual with bladder cancer may face. The answers are to the point and cover the essentials required to make an informed decision for most individuals. For others, a more detailed resource may be required. For helpful sources of additional information see the Appendix.

Each individual's situation is unique. Decisions on treatment may be modified based on the patient's preferences and values and altered by other considerations such as age and coexisting conditions. By becoming an individual knowledgeable of bladder cancer, you will be prepared to fully partner with your physician for your best possible outcome. To your companions and family members, this book will serve to answer the many questions and doubts that may arise. Having your loved ones informed and supportive is a big plus for the individual facing this new challenge.

The book is written in a logical sequence starting with finding a qualified urologist to the basics on bladder cancer, its assessment and treatment. At the end of the book, you will find chapters on complementary medicine, advance care planning, and hospice care. The book can be read in sequence or each chapter can serve as a resource covering the basics of the topic. It is my hope this book will help clarify the many issues and options individuals must face with bladder cancer. For family members, significant others and concerned friends, this resource should help improve your understanding and thus your ability to assist your loved one.

CHAPTER TWO
FINDING A QUALIFIED
UROLOGIST

Understanding bladder cancer is a tremendous first step that will assist you in your treatment. Having a qualified urologist administer the actual treatments and care for you is essential for the best possible outcome. In the following chapter, we will explore what you need to know to assure you have the right urologist.

BESIDES LEARNING ABOUT MY DISEASE, WHAT IS MY MOST IMPORTANT FIRST STEP?

Make sure you have an excellent urologist supervising your care. A urologist is a surgical specialist trained to care for conditions involving the male and female urinary tracts and the male reproductive system. The bladder is part of the urinary system, and a urologist is trained to care for problems involving it, including cancer.

IS IT IMPORTANT TO HAVE A BOARD CERTIFIED UROLOGIST?

A urologist board certified by The American Board of Urology has gone through an accredited urology training program (generally a four year program), following two years of internship and residency in surgery after four years of medical school. The urologist must be in practice after training and provide a detailed list of surgeries, including complications, over a twelve month period. The doctor will then take a two day oral and written test covering a wide spectrum of urology. If he passes, he is certified for a period of ten years. At the end of the ten year period, he must recertify to maintain his board status. Recertification entails a three month surgical and procedure log and a written test as well as reference letters from those in a position to judge the practicing urologist's work. Any malpractice or judgments are also reviewed. Although being board certified does not guarantee you have an excellent urologist, it demonstrates that he has the fund of knowledge to practice urology competently. Even though board certification is voluntary, in today's competitive environment more and more hospitals and insurance plans are requiring their specialists to be certified.

HOW CAN I TELL IF MY UROLOGIST IS BOARD CERTIFIED?

The urologist has worked hard to obtain board certification. The certificate from The American Board of Urology is often displayed openly in his office. If you do not see it, you can simply ask him or you can call 1-866-275-2267 or use this web site: www.certified doctor.org

SHOULD I TRY TO FIND A UROLOGIST WHO HAS BEEN IN PRACTICE FOR YEARS OR A NEWLY TRAINED ONE?

Surgery is a skill which can only be mastered with experience. The saying "practice makes perfect" definitely pertains to surgery. Although a urology training program offers the new physician years of training, his surgical skills will continue to improve with further experience. However, each individual physician has his own innate skills. Some more quickly learn and are simply better at the technical craft of surgery than others. For the most part, urologists finishing an accredited urology program have the training and skill set required to care for patients with bladder cancer.

Experience also counts. As a physician practices the art of medicine, his depth of knowledge and ability to treat grows. Ask your physician how long he has been treating patients with bladder cancer. If you require major surgery ask how many he has performed and if his complication rate matches what is expected.

Physicians by and large do improve as they practice, and all physicians are required to show that they are continuing to learn by partaking in continuing medical education, a requirement to remain licensed. Most physicians are compulsive in their medical practice and care deeply in the care they deliver. They continually strive to improve.

Some physicians may become "burned out" over the years as they continue to face the pressures of a busy medical practice. Similarly, towards the end of a surgeon's career, technical skills may slip due to aging. New urologists are trained in the latest techniques and are familiar with recent medical literature, but may lack practical experience. In the end, recommendations from others and reputation may be your best guide to finding a qualified physician.

WHAT QUALITIES SHOULD MY UROLOGIST HAVE?

Ideally, you should have a competent, technically skilled surgeon who is also approachable and compassionate. You should be able to freely ask questions pertaining to your disease and treatment. Your physician should answer your questions forthrightly. Although some patients prefer a surgeon who will take over all aspects of care with no questions asked, most prefer in depth explanations, especially when alternatives exist and risks are involved.

Your urologist must be an individual who takes your concerns, priorities and values seriously. Your urologist should be a good communicator. It is his responsibility to keep you fully informed of your progress, make you aware immediately if things are not going well, and educate you fully in treatment alternatives. Your specific values should be incorporated into the decision process if alternatives are available. Even if your urologist makes a recommendation and you choose an alternative course (unless you are putting yourself in extreme jeopardy), he should honor your choice and continue his care of you. Becoming an educated patient will make your decision making process easier. Granted, your physician should provide you with the basics, however having time to review and digest the material will allow you to fully understand and accept your treatment regimen, providing you with peace of mind.

Beware of the physician who bombards you with statistics and studies and leaves the decision making to you. After all, you are not a physician and don't have the practical hands on experience he does. Your physician should provide the facts and the statistics, guide you through the information, and make treatment recommendations based on your preferences.

You may find yourself emotionally distraught and overwhelmed. Having a physician on your side is invaluable. You should be able to trust your physician. Complete honesty on the part of your doctor in his care of you is a must. From the doctor's point of view, trust is also a necessity. Physicians have an extremely difficult time dealing with individuals who do not trust them. Without trust, the physician patient relationship is extremely hindered.

Lastly, your urologist should be compassionate. Having cancer is tough enough, you shouldn't have to deal with a rude or arrogant physician. Your urologist should be supportive at all times. He should treat you as an individual and not just as "another cancer patient." People with bladder cancer will require long term follow up and care. Having a compassionate individual to work with will make a tremendous difference

HOW DO I FIND A GOOD BOARD CERTIFIED UROLOGIST?

A good starting point is your primary care physician. He will generally have a number of specialists to whom he generally refers his urology patients. If the primary care physician has been working with these urologists, he should have an appreciation of their skills and temperament. However, this does not mean he is referring you necessarily to the best available urologist in your area. His choices may be limited by insurance or hospital networks. An excellent source of information would be nurses who work in the operating room, recovery room or on the surgical floor where the urologist does his surgery. Asking friends or other individuals who have had experience with the urologist can also prove useful. After a little digging, you can often quickly learn what type of reputation the urologist has in the community.   Generally, if an established urologist has a "good reputation" this is an indication that he has pleased many individuals with his care.

SHOULD I CHECK TO SEE HOW MANY TIMES MY UROLOGIST HAS BEEN SUED?

Given the litigious society we live in, most physicians can face at least one malpractice lawsuit during their careers. In urology, two of the most common causes of litigation would be a surgical mishap leading to a complication, or failure to diagnose cancer in a timely fashion.

Medicine is based on science, but also is an "art." Individuals do not walk into their physicians offices with a diagnosis and treatment plan always readily apparent. Even the best intentioned, thorough physician will make mistakes. Most of these errors do not result in harm. On occasion they do, and a law suit may follow. If a physician develops a good working relationship with a patient, these bad outcomes more often than not are acknowledged and accepted without legal entanglement. Competent, busy physicians may be dealing with a higher mix of complicated patients, leading to a higher number of potential suits. Physicians who have poor "bed side manner" may find themselves dealing with more suits. If a physician has an inordinate number of suits, "red flags" should go up, as competency may be an issue.

For those individuals who wish to check out the malpractice history of their physician, you may request an inquiry from the National Practitioners Data Bank at: 1-800-767-6732 or check the web site: www.npdb-hipdb.com

MY FAMILY WANTS ME TO GO FOR TREATMENT OF MY BLADDER CANCER TO THE "TEACHING HOSPITAL" IN THE CITY. MY LOCAL UROLOGIST IS COMPETENT AND CARING AND I TRUST HIS JUDGEMENT. SHOULD I LISTEN TO MY FAMILY AND SWITCH UROLOGISTS?

As we have discussed in the preceding questions, finding an excellent urologist to partner with is a must. A physician established at a "teaching hospital" (a hospital where physicians are trained in their respective fields of specialty) is at the minimum, competent. A large teaching or academic center would not risk its reputation on an individual who is sub par. Some individuals may be world class surgeons, but not all will be. An individual may be an average surgeon, but a gifted teacher or researcher, making them invaluable to their academic center. Your local community urologist will likely be an individual trained at one of these academic teaching hospitals. In addition, community hospitals also have credentialing and quality review programs to weed out incompetent physicians. In general, it is true the academic center will have more stringent standards and review of their staff. Nevertheless, excellent physicians can be found at the community hospital as well.

ISN'T IT TRUE THAT ACADEMIC OR TEACHING HOSPITALS WILL HAVE THE BEST TECHNOLOGY OR MOST UP TO DATE INFORMATION TO TREAT MY CANCER?

These hospitals generally are at the forefront of innovation regarding technological advances, testing and implementation of new surgical techniques and chemotherapeutic regimens. However, no one center can be excellent in all spheres of medicine. Each will have particular strengths and weaknesses. We are however, fortunate medical knowledge and innovation are shared openly via medical journals and conferences and other means of information exchange. New information and proven effective techniques are rapidly disseminated throughout the medical community. Some teaching hospitals may be "centers of excellence" for a particular procedure or innovative approach that is available at only a few sites in the country. There is naturally a lag time for some procedures to spread to the local level, and if in fact a new procedure carries substantial benefits compared to the standard, and is not available locally, then a referral may be appropriate.

Medical information is scrutinized in journals and reviewed at conferences. The newest treatment regimens for advanced cancer are explored in clinical trials to determine their efficacy and safety. It is only after they are proven that they become adopted as standard practice by most physicians. For the vast majority of individuals with bladder cancer, excellent, comprehensive treatment can be obtained at the local level. For those requiring more specialized care or for those unfortunate individuals with advanced cancer who desire experimental therapy via a clinical trial for their cancer, a referral to the appropriate center may be appropriate.

IF I HAVE MY MAJOR SURGERY PERFORMED AT A TEACHING HOSPITAL, WILL THE ATTENDING PHYSICIAN PERFORM MY SURGERY AND TAKE CARE OF ME AFTERWARDS?

At a teaching hospital, physicians are in training to master their skills before going out into "practice" in their respective fields. Interns are fresh out of medical school with limited practical training. Often they are referred to as PGY 1 (post graduate year 1). Years of training follow (PGY2, PGY3 etc.). Urology residents are required to generally have at least two years of training in a surgical program followed by four years in urology residency. It is the responsibility of the residency director to provide adequate training for these future urologists while assuring patient safety. Practically speaking, there are usually one or more attending physicians who supervise the work of the physicians in training. The attending physicians are board certified, experienced physicians who treat patients while simultaneously training physicians. The residents will be a key component in your care. They will be assessing you both pre- and post-operatively and will be writing orders directing your care. How much of the surgery they get to do is dependent on their years of training and their skills. They will be under the direct supervision of the attending physician. If you have concerns, you should address them with your attending physician.

MY UROLOGIST ALWAYS KEEPS ME WAITING, DOES THIS MEAN HE DOESN'T CARE?

Given the monetary pressures in today's medical practice, some physicians are over booked and cannot see the allotted number of patients scheduled without delays. The theory behind this schedule is the expectation that a number of patients will not show for their appointment, allowing the physician to stay true to the schedule and not fall behind.

However, sometimes all of the patients do show, and the physician is delayed. Even with a carefully thought out schedule, emergencies may arise and some visits unexpectedly take longer than scheduled. The physician wants to devote the time and attention required for each individual. After all, you also expect the same time and attention during your visit. Even the most conscientious physician may find himself running behind in a busy medical practice. This lateness should be recognized by the physician who will often acknowledge it with an apology. If you find it distressing to wait more than fifteen minutes (a reasonable time to wait), you should discuss your feelings with your physician, who often can arrange an appointment at the beginning of the schedule when he will almost be guaranteed to be on time.

WILL THERE BE OTHER PHYSICIANS INVOLVED IN MY TREATMENT OF BLADDER CANCER?

You may need to be referred to an oncologist, a physician specialist in the medical therapy of cancer. At times, a referral to a radiation oncologist, a specialist who treats cancer with radiation, may be required. Other individuals may need to be consulted as well. It is important for your urologist to keep your primary care physician up to date so that he can coordinate your care and if required by your insurance plan, make the appropriate referrals.

CHAPTER THREE
GOING FOR A SECOND OPINION

On a regular basis, magazine articles, books, and television shows implore those with major illnesses to seek out a second opinion. The general consensus is there is much to be gained and little to be lost, so why not seek out a second opinion? The issue certainly is more complicated than generally addressed, and deserves a review. The following chapter provides a second opinion on second opinions.

WHAT ABOUT SECOND OPINIONS?

In general, a competent physician will recommend a second opinion if there is uncertainty regarding your care. This uncertainty could involve the pathology report or debate regarding the most appropriate treatment options. Certainly if the pathology report is in question, a second opinion is mandatory! Your urologist should be able to spell out his treatment plans for you, what to expect and what alternatives may be required, depending on the seriousness of your disease. The plan may change over time as your disease improves or worsens.

You may need a second opinion if you are not doing well and your physician is unable to provide satisfactory explanations and solutions. Occasionally, your urologist may recommend a second opinion if your problem is unusual or particularly complicated. Having a physician you can trust is mandatory when dealing with cancer. Don't let anyone pressure you into a second opinion if you feel confident in your physician's abilities. On the other hand, if you are uncomfortable with your progress or a treatment recommendation, if you are not satisfied with the explanations given to you, don't hesitate to seek out a second opinion. Your urologist should not feel threatened by this request as he wants you to feel comfortable with the plan of action. Only by partnering with your physician can he be most effective.

WILL MY UROLOGIST BE UPSET WHEN I REQUEST A SECOND OPINION?

Many physicians may feel slighted when a patient requests a second opinion. Your urologist may feel somehow you don't trust his explanations, skill, or judgment. On the other hand, when a new patient faces a difficult or unexpected diagnosis, the urologist may find the request not at all unusual. It is important you explain to your urologist why you feel a second opinion is warranted. Urologists are professionals and will graciously facilitate your request. The experienced urologist comes to realize that despite his best efforts, some patients will seek a second opinion. If a patient is particularly concerned or nervous about a proposed treatment regimen, your urologist may welcome your request. Your urologist should facilitate your second opinion by sending appropriate records and telling you whether or not it is necessary for you to bring X rays or pathology slides with you. Your primary care physician may need to be contacted for the referral if your insurance requires it.

WHY DOESN'T MY UROLOGIST WANT ME TO GO FOR A SECOND OPINION?

Often, the urologist may believe the second opinion is unnecessary and will delay treatment. He may be concerned you will not only have a second opinion, but transfer your future care to the urologist providing the second opinion. He may believe that you may get bad advice. It is possible he may feel threatened the next urologist will not agree with his work up or care of you to date.

WHERE DO I FIND A SPECIALIST FOR A SECOND OPINION?

Start by asking your primary care physician. You may be able to see another urologist in your community. Do not see another urologist in the same group as a conflict of interest may deter a different opinion. If you are considering a different course of action, such as radiation or chemotherapy, a referral to the appropriate specialist should be made.

Many times your urologist will be highly supportive and suggest a second opinion. He will offer his recommendations and facilitate your visit to the appropriate physician. If there is an issue regarding the care given at your local hospital, you may wish a referral to a "tertiary" or teaching hospital. In most areas, a referral for this reason is unnecessary, as excellent care is obtainable in the community hospital.

CHAPTER FOUR
BASIC INFORMATION ON
BLADDER CANCER

Cancer unfortunately is a common disease affecting almost all animals. People are equally susceptible; approximately one in three will be afflicted at some time in their life. In this chapter, we will review basic information regarding the bladder, bladder cancer, and cancer in general, including what causes it and some parameters used to determine how serious it is.

WHAT IS THE FUNCTION OF THE BLADDER?

A bladder stores urine and expels it at a convenient time. The bladder is a very useful organ, (tissues working together to accomplish a function), but an individual can live a normal life without one, if required, by surgical creation of a substitute.

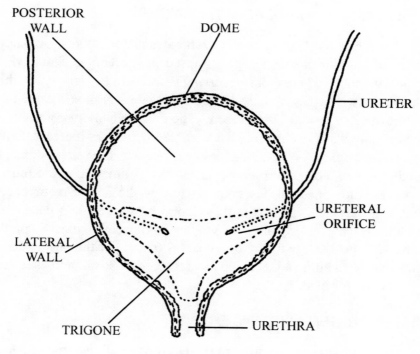

THE BLADDER

ARE THERE DIFFERENT TYPES OF BLADDER CANCER?

More than 90% of bladder cancers arise from the lining bladder cells called transitional cells. Bladder cancer is almost always transitional cell cancer. These cells are also present in the urethra (the body tube which drains the bladder), as well as the renal pelvis (inner lining of the kidneys), and the ureters (the body tube draining the kidneys).

Bladder cancer can vary from the non serious, low grade superficial type (approximately 70%), to the invasive, aggressive type that can spread and prove to be fatal (approximately 30%).

5% of bladder cancer is accounted for by squamous cell carcinoma. This cancer is usually secondary to long term inflammation or infection of the bladder. Even rarer is adenocarcinoma, which accounts for less than 2% of all bladder cancers.

HOW COMMON IS BLADDER CANCER?

The American Cancer Society estimates that in 2006, 61,420 new cases of bladder cancer were diagnosed in the United States with approximately 73% of those occurring in men. In the same year, this cancer caused approximately 13,060 deaths with approximately two out of three of those being in men. The disease is more common in whites than blacks. The incidence of bladder cancer increases with age in both sexes. When bladder cancer occurs in young people, it tends to grow slower and not be as serious. In men, it is the fourth most common cancer. However, because of the rate of recurrences and long term survival, it is the second most prevalent cancer in middle aged and elderly men. In women, it is the eighth most common cancer. The average age at diagnosis is 65. Over the past decade, there has been both an increased incidence, but also an increased rate of survival for bladder cancer [1]

WHAT CAUSED MY CANCER?

A mutation is a disruption in the DNA of a cell, leading to a loss of regulated cell growth. Mutations can occur spontaneously as we age. It is truly amazing that all of us don't develop cancer as we are composed of trillions of cells dividing regularly over decades. Fortunately, our cells have repair mechanisms which can often fix damaged cells before cancer arises. In addition, the immune system can destroy cancer cells before they have a chance to grow into tumors.

Mutations and cancer can also be triggered by environmental factors. Certain chemicals have been identified to be particularly effective at inducing mutations in our DNA and subsequent cancer. These chemicals are called carcinogens. Smoking is the most common culprit! Cigarette smoking has a strong link with bladder cancer. Studies have shown approximately 50% of bladder cancer is secondary to tobacco smoke. Smoking releases dozens of carcinogens into the lungs and then into the blood stream. Many of

---

[1]   National Cancer Institute SEER Cancer Statistics Review 1973-1997. Available at: http://seer.cancer.gov/Publications/CSR 1973-1997/bladder/pdf.

these carcinogens are excreted by the kidneys. After years of being exposed to this toxic soup, a smoker's bladder has a much greater chance of developing bladder cancer, two to three times, and in heavy smokers up to five times the rate compared to those people who have never smoked. The risk clearly correlates with the number of years the individual has smoked and the number of cigarettes smoked per year. Fortunately, after you stop smoking, your risk gradually decreases. Once you develop bladder cancer, it is mandatory to stop smoking. It is now known failure to stop smoking leads to a much worse outcome compared to those with bladder cancer that stop smoking.[2]

IT IS TOO DIFFICULT TO QUIT SMOKING; IS THERE ANY SURE FIRE WAY TO QUIT?

Tobacco smoke contains nicotine, an extremely addictive chemical. Men overall find it easier to quit smoking than women. When facing the prospects of losing your bladder to cancer or possibly your life, most individuals will become convinced and many simply stop smoking "cold turkey." Unfortunately, many choose not to quit until their cancer repeatedly recurs or becomes invasive, needlessly placing their health at risk. For those who need assistance in quitting, nicotine patches, gum, and lozenges are all available over the counter. These products allow the smoker to quit without experiencing the discomfort of withdrawal from nicotine. Many smokers also find hypnosis or support groups useful. In addition, prescription medication is available.

ARE THERE ANY OTHER KNOWN CAUSES?

Occupational exposure may account for up to 20% of bladder cancers. Those exposed to aniline dyes (used to color fabrics), aldehydes (used in chemical dyes and in the rubber and textile industries) and those using organic chemicals (used in a wide range of

---

[2]   Fleshner N., Moadel A, Herr H, et al. Influence of smoking status on outcomes in patients with tobacco-associated superficial transitional cell carcinoma (TCC) of the bladder. J Urol. 1999; 16 (4suppl):172. Abstract 664.

occupations) are all at increased risk. Individuals previously treated with radiation to the pelvis or having received cyclophosphamide (a type of chemotherapy) are at markedly increased risk for developing bladder cancer. If your well water is high in arsenic, your risk may also be increased. Studies have also correlated obesity and a high fat diet, especially with increased cholesterol, as a possible contributing factor.

CAN I HELP TO PREVENT BLADDER CANCER BY DRINKING MORE FLUIDS?

Surprisingly, the answer may be yes. In a recent study, the relationship of diet to cancer was analyzed in a group of 47,000 health professionals.[3] In the case of bladder cancer, those who drank the most fluid (greater than 10 cups/day) had half the risk as those who drank the least (less than 5 cups/day). The type of nonalcoholic beverage was less important than the total amount.

WILL MY CHILDREN BE AT HIGHER RISK OF DEVELOPING BLADDER CANCER?

Although there have been clusters of bladder cancer reported, most researchers believe these may be secondary to risk factors such as smoking and exposure to carcinogens. At this time, there is no convincing evidence bladder cancer risk is hereditary. If an environmental factor caused your cancer and your children are exposed as well, their risk of cancer may be increased.

WHAT IS CANCER?

The basic building block of the body is the cell. Cells are specialized to perform a particular function. Skin cells are distinctly different from liver cells which are different from bladder cells. An organ is composed of various cells working in unison to carry out a body function. Cells eventually get old and die. New cells are created by cell division. When cells are behaving normally,

---

[3] Michaud DS, Spiegelman D,Clinton SK et al. Fluid intake and the risk of bladder cancer in men. N Eng J Med. 1999;340(18): 1390-1397

they only generate enough new cells to replace the old dying ones. Occasionally, cell growth becomes unchecked. As the cells continue to divide, a tumor (abnormal growth of cells) may form. Such tumors may be benign (no ability to spread beyond their organ of origin) or cancerous (a malignant tumor with the ability to spread beyond their organ of origin and cause harm and possibly death).

Cell growth is closely regulated by genes which are composed of DNA located in the command center of the cell, the nucleus. When the genes become defective, cell growth can become unregulated, and tumors can develop. Oncogenes, also called cancer genes, can be activated, resulting in uncontrolled cell growth. Other genes which help prevent abnormal cell growth called tumor suppressor genes may be inactivated. Genes can be activated which enhance the tumor cell's ability to spread throughout the body. The body's immune system is a critical safeguard against the formation of cancerous tumors, often destroying the abnormal cells before they have a chance to grow and divide.

HOW DOES CANCER SPREAD?

Cancer cells can spread throughout the body. They can spread through the lymphatic system, composed of lymph channels and lymph nodes, or distantly to other organs or the skeleton via the blood stream (hematogenous spread). In the case of bladder cancer, the cells can also spread by being carried in the urine and implanting in other locations in the urinary tract.

HOW CAN I TELL IF MY BLADDER CANCER IS LIKELY TO SPREAD?

Larger tumors are more likely to spread than smaller tumors. Another critical concern is the grade of the tumor. Normal cells are specialized, differentiated to perform specific function, and have a typical structural arrangement with surrounding cells. As cancers worsen, the cells become less specialized, less differentiated, and lose their normal structural arrangement, resulting in a higher pathologic grade.

In the case of bladder cancer, pathologists classify them into 3 grades based on a number of criteria:

Grade 1: low grade, well differentiated

Grade 2: intermediate grade, moderately differentiated

Grade 3: high grade, poorly differentiated

The higher grade tumors have a greater propensity to metastasize-spread throughout the body.

For bladder cancer, another key indicator for likelihood to spread is the depth of penetration into the bladder wall. The bladder wall is composed of an inner lining called the urothelium (made up of transitional cells) which rests on a membrane layer called the basement membrane, below which is the connective tissue layer (support tissues) called the lamina propria. Within the lamina propria lies a small amount of muscle called the muscularis mucosa. Deep to the lamina propria is the deep muscle of the bladder arranged in three layers. This layer is called the muscularis propria. Tumors located in the inside, superficial layers of the bladder wall are unlikely to spread. Tumors that grow into the deeper layers (down into the muscle of the bladder wall) are much more likely to spread. Furthermore, there is a definite link between the grade of the tumor and its likelihood of invasion. Low grade tumors are almost always noninvasive, while high grade tumors are usually invasive. In general, papillary tumors, which are delicate and frond like in appearance are usually low grade and superficial. This is to be contrasted to sessile tumors which appear solid, are often high grade and invasive. Depth of invasion is critical in establishing prognosis. The tumor which invades into the lamina propria is a far more serious tumor than the superficial tumor which demonstrates no invasion. It has a much higher propensity to progress to the muscle invasive tumor, a much more dangerous cancer, with a high risk for spreading beyond the bladder. For further information see Chapter 6.

SUPERFICIAL
PAPILLARY
TUMOR

FROND LIKE
APPEARANCE

BLADDER
WALL

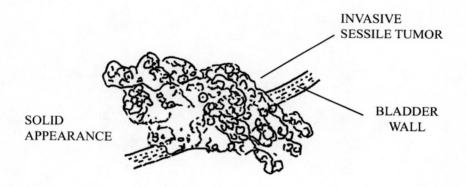

INVASIVE
SESSILE TUMOR

BLADDER
WALL

SOLID
APPEARANCE

HOW IS THE GRADE OF CANCER DETERMINED?

The pathologist studies the prepared slides and makes a determination of the grade of cancer. There are a number of criterions that are used: degree of cellularity, nuclear crowding, loss of polarity and differentiation, nuclear pleomorphism, chromatin pattern and mitotic activity. In layman's terms, the pathologist looks at the size, shape and relationship of the cancer cells. The nucleus is often abnormal since it contains damaged or mutated DNA. Cancer cells look different than normal cells. The greater the difference from normal, the higher the grade will be. These parameters are utilized to reduce the subjective nature of pathology. In the end, the pathologist assigns a grade. Since grading is actually a continuum, many pathologists find that by adding "½" to the grading scale, they can more accurately grade what they are seeing:

Grade 1, Grade 1 ½, Grade 2, Grade 2 ½, Grade 3.

Because pathology is somewhat subjective, it is not unusual to have a difference of opinion on the final grade of a cancer by individual pathologists. Additionally, a specific tumor may have multiple grades within it. The pathologist may report the spectrum of grades such as grade 1-2 or report the highest, most dangerous grade. If there are multiple tumors in the same bladder, their individual grades may vary.

CHAPTER FIVE
INITIAL EVALUATION

The medical history of those with bladder cancer varies. For many patients, the first clue is blood in the urine, while in others, it may be an alteration in urination. Sometimes a tumor is found inadvertently on an X ray or ultrasound exam. In all cases, an initial assessment is implemented by the urologist. In this chapter, we will review the presenting findings of those with bladder cancer and how they are initially "worked up."

WHAT IS THE DIFFERENCE BETWEEN A SIGN AND A SYMPTOM?

A sign is a physical finding from an underlying disease or disorder which can be noted by the individual or the physician. A symptom is something the individual feels or experiences from a disease. A clinical sign is a physical finding, while a symptom is something the individual experiences.

I PASSED SOME BLOOD IN MY URINE SEVERAL WEEKS AGO, THERE WASN'T ANY PAIN AND IT HASN'T OCCURRED AGAIN, IS THIS SOMETHING I NEED TO BE CONCERNED ABOUT?

Absolutely! Approximately three quarters of individuals with bladder cancer initially present with blood in their urine. The blood may be visible to the naked eye (gross hematuria), or seen with a microscope only (microscopic hematuria). In the case of gross hematuria secondary to bladder cancer, it is often total (throughout the entire stream) and may be intermittent. Generally, there is no pain associated with it. I have seen many patients over the years who had gross hematuria months earlier who falsely assumed their condition was not serious since the bleeding stopped and there was no pain, only to come in later with recurrent bleeding, their tumors needlessly more advanced. When an individual experiences gross hematuria, a work up is a must! Gross hematuria at times can become quite severe to the point blood clots can restrict the flow of urine. What could have been an elective assessment then becomes a mad dash to the emergency room for catheterization (passing a tube into the bladder) and irrigation or an emergency procedure. Of course, there are other causes for gross hematuria, such as urinary infections, kidney stones or tumors in the kidney, all of which require assessment.

MY PHYSICIAN FOUND A SMALL AMOUNT OF BLOOD ON A URINE DIPSTICK DURING ROUTINE EXAM, IS THERE ANY NEED TO FOLLOW THIS?

If a urine dipstick is positive for blood, it is recommended to check the urine under a microscope. The urine is first spun down to separate out the sediment and is then examined under the high power lens. If there are more than 3 red blood cells per high power field it is felt to be significant. If there are no other reasons for the presence of blood such as a urinary infection, the urine should be rechecked. If there is a persistent presence of significant microscopic hematuria, an assessment is recommended. When there is a large amount of microscopic hematuria, especially in older individuals with risk factors for bladder cancer, there is no need to repeat the urinalysis as a workup should be done.

IS ASYMPTOMATIC MICROSCOPIC HEMATURIA ALWAYS A SIGN OF SOMETHING SERIOUS?

A small amount of microscopic hematuria in an individual without symptoms (asymptomatic microscopic hematuria) can be found in many healthy individuals. It has been estimated that up to 10% of the population has asymptomatic microscopic hematuria. In brief, the older you are (generally over the age of 40), the more risk factors you have (smoking, occupational exposure), and the more red blood cells present, the more likely serious pathology (disease of the urinary tract including bladder cancer) will be found. If you have persistent microscopic hematuria without a known cause, a urologic assessment is recommended.

WHAT IS THE WORK UP FOR HEMATURIA?

When assessment for hematuria is required, the entire urinary tract is evaluated. This is accomplished via imaging studies (X ray or ultrasound), cystoscopy (visual inspection of the bladder), and possibly cytology (urine test for cancer cells). There are multiple causes for blood in the urine, including the possibility of kidney disease, kidney, ureteral or bladder stones, infection, or enlargement of the prostate.

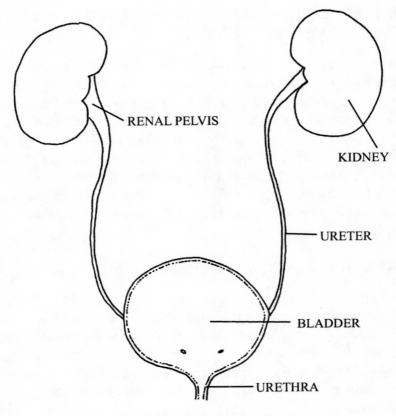

RENAL PELVIS

KIDNEY

URETER

BLADDER

URETHRA

THE URINARY TRACT

I HAVE BEEN EXPERIENCING BURNING WHEN I URINATE, BUT MY PRIMARY CARE PHYSICIAN DIDN'T FIND AN INFECTION, DO I REALLY NEED TO BE REFERRED TO A UROLOGIST?

Approximately twenty percent of patients with bladder cancer will complain of irritative voiding symptoms. These symptoms include urinary urgency (a need to rush to the bathroom), burning and urinary frequency. These same symptoms are present in other urologic conditions such as infection, bladder instability and prostatic enlargement in men. These symptoms are most commonly associated with a diffuse superficial form of transitional cell cancer of the bladder called CIS (carcinoma in situ). Unfortunately for some, their diagnosis may be delayed since these symptoms are present in so many other diseases.

It is important to be assessed for persistent irritative symptoms!

MY UROLOGIST HAS RECOMMENDED A CYSTOSCOPY. IS THIS REALLY NECESSARY?

Cystoscopy (examination of the bladder) is usually the first step in making the diagnosis of bladder cancer. Given the signs and symptoms suggesting bladder cancer, or an X ray or ultrasound revealing a possible bladder tumor, cystoscopy is a must. Cystoscopy can be accomplished with either a flexible cystoscope or a rigid scope. The flexible cystoscope is composed of small optical fibers encased by a plastic sheath. A rigid scope has glass lenses within a metal sheath. Both cystoscopes are passed directly through the urethra into the bladder to visualize the inside surface. Cystoscopy can be accomplished in both the urologist's office or as an outpatient at a hospital or surgicenter.

MY UROLOGIST SAYS HE CAN DO FLEXIBLE CYSTOSCOPY RIGHT IN HIS OFFICE. WILL I HAVE TERRIBLE PAIN DURING THE EXAM?

The flexible cystoscope is easier and less painful to pass, especially for males whose urethra is longer and more tortuous than in females. Flexible cystoscopy is readily accomplished in the doctor's office. A lubricant is applied to the scope to ease passage. Local anesthesia can be squirted into the urethra prior to passing the scope. Discomfort from the cystoscope is usually well tolerated and short in duration. The discomfort usually lasts a few seconds as the scope is passed through the prostate. At that time, you may feel a pressure sensation. In females, passage of the scope is quick and relatively painless.

During the exam, your bladder will be filled with sterile water to allow complete visualization of all the surfaces. You may feel like you have to urinate. During flexible cystoscopy, small biopsies can be obtained. Any bleeding from the biopsy site is readily controlled. The biopsy and cauterization will cause pain for a few seconds. A mild oral sedative can be taken prior to an exam, but is generally not necessary. An entire examination may take only a few minutes. If biopsies are done, the exam will be a little longer. Flexible cystoscopy is very convenient. You can drive yourself to and from the office. After the exam, you can generally go right back to work. If a tumor is found that is too large to treat with a flexible cystoscope, you will be scheduled for an additional procedure at a hospital or surgicenter.

MY UROLOGIST HAS SCHEDULED ME FOR RIGID CYSTOSCOPY AT THE SURGICENTER, WHAT CAN I EXPECT?

The rigid cystoscope, although easy to pass in a female is difficult to pass without sedation in a male. The rigid cystoscope allows for generous biopsy specimens and removal of small tumors. Cystoscopy therefore can provide for both diagnosis and treatment at the same time. If a large cancer is found, removal with a resectoscope can be used to remove it at the same time. If multiple biopsies or resection of a cancer is done, spinal or general anesthesia may be required. Since rigid cystoscopy generally causes more discomfort than flexible cystoscopy and requires more anesthetic, you can expect to be out of work at least one day. In addition, someone will need to drive you home from the surgicenter or hospital.

HOW DOES THE UROLOGIST DECIDE ON WHETHER TO DO FLEXIBLE OR RIGID CYSTOSCOPY?

If you are being initially screened for asymptomatic microscopic hematuria, a urologist will often choose flexible cystoscopy as the first step. He is not certain whether or not you have a bladder cancer or other condition causing the hematuria. Flexible cystoscopy will provide that answer in a less time consuming, less painful and more cost effective way than rigid cystoscopy. On the other hand, if there is a high likelihood a tumor is present, it makes sense to do rigid cystoscopy and if required, resection all at one setting. If you are experiencing gross hematuria, flexible cystoscopy does not provide adequate visualization, and rigid cystoscopy is warranted. Many urologists use both types of cystoscopes, but some do not have the flexible cystoscope in their office.

MY UROLOGIST SAYS I CAN WATCH THE ENTIRE PROCEDURE ON A VIDEO SCREEN. I'M A LITTLE SQUEAMISH. SHOULD I WATCH?

The cystoscope may be attached to a camera so images appear on a video screen. This technology will allow your urologist to actually show you the findings during the examination. I have found many patients are at first hesitant to "view their insides," but later thank me afterwards for having the opportunity. They often view the images with fascination and curiosity.

DO I NEED TO DO ANYTHING SPECIAL AFTER CYSTOSCOPY?

After cystoscopy, you should drink plenty of water, especially if there is some bleeding present. Mild discomfort generally lasts approximately 24 hours. It is not unusual to have some bleeding after cystoscopy, which is often the case if biopsies have been done. If you have had biopsies or a tumor has been resected, your urologist should give you specific instructions on what to avoid. Generally, it is best not to partake in heavy exercise or exertion. Avoid getting constipated as straining can start bleeding. You should call your urologist if you have persistent or severe pain afterwards, heavy bleeding (dark bloody urine or clots), persistent bleeding lasting more than a few days, inability to urinate, or a fever (temperature greater than 100 degrees Fahrenheit).

CAN CYTOLOGY BE USED INSTEAD OF CYSTOSCOPY TO RULE OUT BLADDER CANCER?

Urinary cytology is the examination of urine using special stains to look for cancer cells. These cells would have been those that have broken off (exfoliated) from the lining of the urinary tract. Voided urine is sent for analysis. First voided morning urine should not be used as there is a higher rate of cellular degeneration. To enhance the yield of cells, the bladder can be barbotaged (flushed). Cytology is most useful for high grade or aggressive tumors and for those with carcinoma in situ (CIS). In low to intermediate grade tumors, cytology may not be positive because these tumors may not exfoliate cells into the urine. In addition, if low grade tumor cells are exfoliated, they may appear to the pathologist to be identical to normal bladder cells. Due to the limitations of sensitivity of cytology, it is not a very good screening test, but proves to be valuable in following some individuals who have already been diagnosed and treated for bladder cancer.

Because a positive cytology is very specific for cancer, it is highly predictive of transitional cell cancer even if no tumor is visible during cystoscopy. Additional information can be obtained with urine cytology. The DNA content and measurement of the amount of abnormal DNA can be determined. In general, as the amount of abnormal DNA is increased, the prognosis is worsened.

ARE THERE ANY OTHER URINE TESTS THAT ARE HELPFUL IN MAKING THE DIAGNOSIS?

There has been continued research and a subsequent array of urine tests to screen for bladder cancer. Some of these newer tests include:

Bladder Tumor Antigen (BTA): measures basement membrane protein antigen released into the urine, a protein from the bladder wall.

NMP22: measures nuclear matrix protein 22

Aura Teck FDP: measures fibrin, fibrinogen degradation products

Telomerase: measures the enzyme used to preserve telomeres (the ends of chromosomes required to continue cell division)

Hyaluronic Acid, Hyaluronidase: substances which have a role in blood vessel growth in bladder tumors and tumor progression. [1]

Research goes on and newer tests may prove to be both more sensitive (positive if cancer is present) and more specific (not positive for other reasons). At this time, none of the urine tests are sensitive enough to take the place of cystoscopy in the initial evaluation of an individual suspected to have bladder cancer. In general, cytology as

---

[1]   Ehab A. El-Gabry, Stephen E. Strup, Leonard G. Gomella, AUA Update Series, Volume 19, Lesson 19, 147-148, American Urological Association, Inc. 2000.

an adjunct to cystoscopy is more helpful than any of the urine bladder cancer tests to date.

AS PART OF MY INITIAL WORK UP, MY PHYSICIAN HAS ORDERED A CAT SCAN. WHAT'S THE PURPOSE AND ARE THERE ANY ALTERNATIVES?

When an individual has gross hematuria or persistent microscopic hematuria, a complete assessment of the urinary tract is required. Although cystoscopy is the test of choice for examination of the bladder, imaging studies are required to make sure there is no disease in the upper tracts (kidneys and ureters). Bleeding can be caused from many different disorders including transitional cell carcinoma of the upper tracts, kidney or ureteral stones, or renal cell carcinoma (cancer of the parenchyma or fleshy part of the kidneys). Your urologist has a number of options to choose from. There are advantages and disadvantages of each.

Intravenous pyelogram (IVP) is accomplished by injecting a contrast agent into your vein and then obtaining X ray images. The contrast is excreted by your kidneys, subsequently filling the lumen of the kidneys, ureters and the bladder. The contrast allows one to see subtle filling defects within chambers of the urinary tract, possibly representing tumor, stone or blood clot. Tumors of the fleshy part of the kidneys can also be seen. The study also allows for an assessment of renal function. It is a sensitive test for renal obstruction, which can occur because of cancer. Disadvantages of the study include the possibility of an IV contrast agent allergy, which occasionally may be serious.

You will be asked whether you have a sea food allergy, a known allergy to iodine or to IV contrast. If this is the case, you may need to be premedicated prior to the exam to avoid a reaction. Although the study is quite useful at visualizing the upper tracts, it is not very good at picking up subtle tumors on the bladder surface. If your kidneys do not function well (you have renal insufficiency), the contrast may cause harm to your kidneys and the imaging will not be as good. For pregnant women, any X ray exam could be potentially damaging to the fetus and therefore, will not be performed.

Ultrasonography can check for a kidney tumor, stone, or obstruction. Bladders filled with urine can be scanned. There is no contrast or X rays involved, and therefore the study can be accomplished in those with renal disease, contrast allergies or for women who are pregnant. Although larger tumors of the bladder are often visible, it is not a good study to rule out urothelial cancer (transitional cell cancer of the urinary tract lining) since smaller tumors or flat tumors in the lining are not visible. Also, other conditions such as enlarged folds in the bladder or enlarged prostates can be confused with bladder tumors. Ultrasound exams are generally fast, painless, and relatively inexpensive. An ultrasound combined with cystoscopy plus cytology (to rule out cancer cells) is a reasonable assessment for those with a low likelihood of having upper tract disease.

CT Scan or CAT (computerized axial tomography) provides a computerized cross sectional visualization of the abdomen and pelvis. X ray images are synthesized into exquisitely detailed images. The CT scan can be done with or without IV contrast, and therefore has the same limitations as IVP in those with allergies to contrast or renal insufficiency. These studies are excellent for finding renal cell cancers and stones within the kidneys and ureter, but not very good at delineating cancers of the lining. CT scan is often an important part of staging bladder cancer, determining whether the cancer has spread.

Magnetic Resonance Imaging (MRI) is a technology which uses strong magnets to provide detailed images of your internal organs. Like ultrasound, this study has no known harmful effects on the body. It does not require contrast injection like CT scan and can be done safely in patients with renal insufficiency. It is not generally used for initial screening. Many individuals find the test uncomfortable due to a loud noise heard throughout the test, in addition to the close quarters the machine requires, leading to feelings of claustrophobia. A mild sedative may be required if the test is necessary and the individual experiences these uncomfortable feelings.

Retrograde Pyelography is a contrast study of the ureters and renal collecting system done during rigid cystoscopy. The urologist injects contrast up the ureters through their respective openings in the bladder. X rays can be done during the injection and captured on film. Retrograde pyelography is often required if there is an uncertain abnormal finding on a preliminary IVP or CT scan. Visualization of the ureters and renal collecting systems is superior to images on IVP or CT scan. The retrograde study can be followed by biopsy or even direct visualization of the ureter or renal lining with a ureteroscope if warranted.

CHAPTER SIX
STAGING OF BLADDER CANCER

Initial treatment may eradicate an individual's bladder cancer, however, for many, recurrent tumors may develop. Up to 70% of individuals will have recurrent bladder cancer after initial therapy. In approximately one third of patients, not only will tumors recur, but they will become more serious over time, developing a higher grade or stage. This chapter will review the importance of staging bladder cancer, the single most important predictor of future problems. In addition, we will review other important indicators that impact the prognosis.

After the diagnosis of cancer is made, it is critical to establish the stage of the cancer. Cancer stage quantifies the extent of cancer in the individual. The number of tumors, their size, whether or not they have grown into the wall of the organ or spread beyond, all fit into the various stages of a particular cancer. Most cancers can be found at an early, nonlethal stage. As they grow and worsen, they can invade the wall of the organ they lodge in, spread locally through the organ into surrounding tissue, or spread throughout the body via the lymphatic or blood system.

In the case of bladder cancer, initial stage is critical in predicting the prognosis. For individuals with bladder cancer, recurrence (repeated tumors) is common. For many, progression (the development of higher grade, invasive or metastatic cancer) is also a real concern. By looking at the initial stage of the bladder cancer and restaging with each new cancer recurrence, the urologist can predict or prognosticate the possibility of the individual developing more life threatening invasive disease which has the ability to spread beyond the bladder and lead to death. Treatment options exist at each stage of cancer. It is the goal of the urologist to preserve your bladder as long as possible without jeopardizing your life with a cancer that may spread and become incurable.

HOW CLOSELY IS STAGE LINKED WITH SURVIVAL?

There is a very close relationship between survival of an individual and the stage of bladder cancer at diagnosis. For superficial disease, five year survival rates are greater than 90%. Once the cancer has spread into the bladder muscle and beyond, survival is markedly reduced. Five year survival in those with T2 disease (tumor invading superficial bladder muscle) is 60-75%, T3 disease (tumor invading deep muscle) 36-58%, and for those with T4 disease (tumor invading surrounding organs) or with node positive disease, 4-35%.[1] With distant (metastatic) spread, survival at five years is less than 5%.

HOW IS THE INITIAL STAGE DETERMINED?

Most individuals with bladder cancer will undergo an initial removal of their bladder tumor by biopsy or for larger tumors by resection of their tumor via a resectoscope. For complete details see Chapter 8. Once this tumor is removed, the pathologist will determine and report on the extent of tumor invasion into the wall of the bladder. If the tumor has grown into the prostate, tissue removal via the resectoscope from this location will also be reviewed and reported pathologically. This pathologic diagnosis determines the initial stage of the cancer.

---

[1] Stein, J.P., Lieskovsky, G., Cote, R., Groshen, S., Feng, A.C., Boyd, S. et al: Radical cystectomy in the treatment of invasive bladder cancer: long-term results in 1,054 patients. J Clin Oncol, 19:2425, 2003.

WHAT OTHER MEANS ARE USED TO ESTABLISH STAGE?

When dealing with large tumors after the initial cancer resection, your urologist may do a manual exam under anesthesia. By pressing deeply on the pelvis, the urologist may be able to palpate the tumor and assess its possible spread beyond the bladder. With modern technology and the availability of the CT scan, the manual exam is now of less importance. The CT scan can often visualize a thickened or distorted bladder wall, indicating the possibility of tumor involvement or extension through the wall. More importantly, it can determine spread to adjacent organs or lymph node involvement. Distant spread into the abdomen or beyond may also be seen. Other studies, such as the Bone Scan or Chest X ray can assess the presence and extent of metastatic diseases. MRI can be used for those with limited kidney function that cannot have a CT scan. More recently, Positron Emission Tomography (PET) scan has become available. This study can sometimes locate small deposits of metastatic disease not visible on CT or MRI scan.

CAN YOU EXPLAIN THE MOST COMMON STAGING SYSTEM FOR BLADDER CANCER?

The TNM system is most widely used. This system classifies the extent of cancer by looking at three components: the Primary Tumor (T), Lymph Node involvement (N) and Distant Metastasis(M).

Primary Tumor (T)

TX	Primary tumor cannot be assessed
TO	No evidence of primary tumor
Tis	Carcinoma in situ: "flat tumor"
Ta	Noninvasive papillary carcinoma
T1	Tumor invades subepithelial connective tissue
T2	Tumor invades superficial muscle (inner half)
T3a	Tumor invades deep muscle (outer half)
T3b	Tumor invades deep muscle or perivesicle fat

T4 Tumor invades any of the following: prostate, uterus vagina, pelvic wall, abdominal wall

T4a Tumor invades prostate, uterus or vagina

T4b Tumor invades pelvic wall or abdominal wall

LYMPH NODE (N)

NX Regional lymph nodes cannot be assessed

N0 No regional lymph node metastasis

N1 Metastasis in a single lymph node, 2 cm or less in greatest dimension

N2 Metastasis in a single lymph node more than 2 cm but not more than 5 cm in greatest dimension, or multiple lymph nodes, none more than 5 cm in greatest dimension

N3 Metastasis in a lymph node more than 5 cm in greatest dimension

DISTANT METASTASIS (M)

MX Presence of distant metastasis cannot be assessed

M0 No distant metastasis

M1 Distant metastasis

HOW ACCURATE IS BLADDER CANCER STAGING?

For many, the cancer may be actually understaged, the actual extent of disease is worse than the stage that has been determined. Errors can occur in the initial tumor resection. Muscle invasion can be "missed" by an incomplete resection or by sampling error in the preparation of pathology slides or in the interpretation by the pathologist. In addition, metastatic disease cannot be picked up with imaging studies such as CT scan in the early stages of spread, but only after the cancer has grown enough to cause lymph node enlargement or new tumors in distant locations. Microscopic disease outside the bladder cannot be imaged.

BESIDES SUPERFICIAL BLADDER CANCER, MY UROLOGIST FOUND SOME TRANSITIONAL CELL CANCER IN MY PROSTATE. DOES THIS FINDING MAKE MY STAGE WORSE?

It may or may not. Since bladder cancer can implant "downstream," it is not uncommon for bladder cancer located near the bladder neck (the opening of the bladder into the prostatic urethra) to eventually show up in the prostatic fossa. Although the original TNM classification for bladder cancer would classify prostate invasion as a stage T4a, a closer examination of primary transitional cell cancer of the prostate is available to more accurately differentiate the extent of involvement in the prostate.

Similar to the classification in the bladder, prostatic involvement is stratified by the depth of involvement:

Tis	pu	Carcinoma in situ, involvement of the prostatic urethra
Tis	pd	Carcinoma in situ, involvement of the prostatic ducts
T1		Tumor invades subepithelial connective tissue
T2		Tumor invades any of the following: prostatic stroma, corpus spongiosum, periurethral muscle
T3		Tumor invades any of the following: corpus cavernosum beyond prostatic capsule, bladder neck
T4		Tumor invades other adjacent organs (invasion of bladder)

Primary transitional cell cancer of the prostate without bladder cancer is usually serious, with more than 50% having T3 or T4 disease and approximately 20% having distant spread.[2] When bladder cancer is present, many patients will eventually develop superficial involvement of the prostate after the urothelium becomes involved with CIS. Superficial involvement of the prostate including

---

[2]   Epstein, J.I. Pathology of Prostatic Neoplasia. Campbell's Urology,Volume 4 2002; 3033.

ductal involvement will not worsen the prognosis and is amenable to local therapy. Generally, higher stage bladder cancers are more likely to develop invasive disease in the prostate. If invasive stromal involvement is found in the prostate, the prognosis is markedly worsened even if the primary bladder cancer is low grade, noninvasive disease. However, minimal stromal invasion will not likely be as serious as more extensive involvement of the stroma.

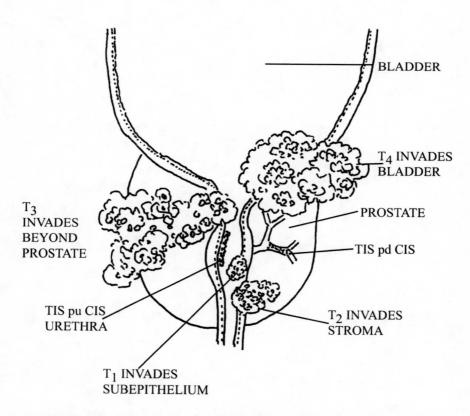

PROSTATIC INVOLVEMENT BY TRANSITIONAL CELL CARCINOMA

IS THE GRADE OF CANCER PART OF THE STAGE?

Although the tumor grade is a very important prognostic indicator, it is not part of the stage of the cancer, which reflects the extent of the cancer. The grade and stage of bladder cancer are however, closely linked. Low grade cancers are rarely invasive, while high grade cancers are rarely superficial. If a high grade cancer is reported to be superficial, sampling error is often at fault and repeat biopsy or resection may be called for.

CHAPTER SEVEN
NATURAL HISTORY OF
SUPERFICIAL BLADDER
CANCER

Once an individual develops bladder cancer, there is a high likelihood that even after removal of the cancer, recurrence will occur. Depending on the initial presentation, some 60-90% will at some time experience recurrent disease. Due to the high recurrence rate, bladder cancer is the second most prevalent cancer in middle aged and elderly men. Recurrence requires repeated endeavors at tumor removal and the possibility of adding other treatment regimens, which can be time consuming, costly and emotionally and physically challenging.

In some individuals recurrence is also accompanied by progression, the development of higher grade, invasive bladder cancer with the propensity to spread and possibly take the life of the individual. For many individuals with low stage, low grade disease, recurrences may be minimal and progression almost nil. For those with more intermediate grade and stage, there exists a higher recurrence and progression rate.

The urologist must vigilantly follow those at risk. Treatment regimens and surveillance exams are altered based on the clinical progress each individual makes. The urologist's goal is to preserve the patient's bladder as long as his life is not being threatened by bladder cancer. Understanding the natural history of the various stages of superficial bladder cancer is critical in formulating an appropriate surveillance and treatment regimen.

WHAT IS THE PROGNOSIS FOR THE VARIOUS STAGES OF BLADDER CANCER?

In the case of bladder cancer, the seriousness of the disease varies widely by stage. Cancer stage is the most important prognostic indicator. In general, the lower stages have fewer propensities to progress to the more serious, potentially life threatening invasive cancer which can spread and become incurable. Unfortunately, some individuals may first present with invasive or metastatic bladder cancer, already too advanced to be cured.

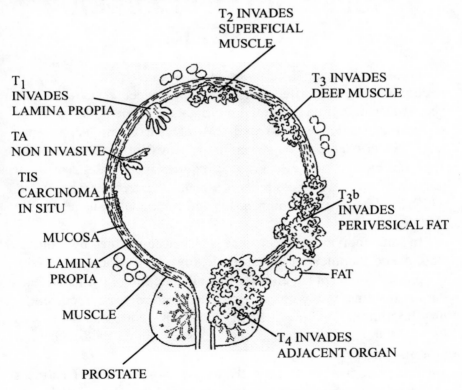

STAGING DIAGRAM BLADDER CANCER

Carcinoma in situ (CIS or Tis): although these "flat" tumors are confined to the most superficial layer, they are generally multi-focal, high grade and have a high likelihood of invasion with a substantial risk for cancer death. They may appear as red velvety or granular areas, or may not be visible through the cystoscope, but are found on random biopsy. CIS will usually result in an abnormal cytology. If an individual has diffuse CIS with irritative symptoms, progression to invasive disease can be expected in up to 80%. For those with only focal CIS, without symptoms, progression occurs in less than 10%. In a recent series from the Mayo Clinic, the rate of progression per year was 4%[1]. When CIS is associated with even low grade, early stage bladder cancers, progression is seen in over 80%, similar to those with diffuse, symptomatic CIS. When CIS is found in conjunction with superficial bladder cancer, the prognosis is markedly worsened.

Ta lesions: these tumors are papillary in appearance (having delicate, flimsy fronds), are generally low grade, and have low rates of progression to more serious cancer. They account for approximately 70% of superficial bladder cancers. The urothelium lacks capillaries and lymphatics, and therefore these tumors almost always remain localized. In one study, only 4% developed progression to muscle invasive or metastatic disease over 39 months.[2]

T1 lesions: these tumors can be papillary or nodular in appearance. These tumors invade through the basement membrane into the connective tissue layer (lamina propria). This layer has both lymphatics and capillaries, and therefore these tumors have a higher propensity to spread compared to Ta tumors. They are more aggressive and generally have a higher grade than Ta lesions. In the same study sited above for Ta tumors, the progression rate for T1 tumors was 30%.[3]

---

[1]   Cheng L, Cheville JC, Neumann RM, et al. Survival of patients with carcinoma in situ of the urinary bladder. Cancer. 1999; 85(11): 2469-2474.

[2]   Jewett H, King L, Shelley W: A study of 365 cases of infiltrating bladder cancer: Relationship of certain pathological characteristics to prognosis after extirpation. J Urol 1964; 92: 668-678.

[3]   Jewett H, King L, Shelley W: A study of 365 cases of infiltrating bladder cancer: Relationship of certain pathological characteristics to prognosis after extirpation. J Urol 1964; 92: 668-678.

T2 lesions: tumors in this stage have superficially invaded the muscularis propria, the thick muscle layer of the bladder. These tumors usually are high grade. Although they may be amenable to local therapy, they have a high rate of further invasion and are at high risk for developing metastatic disease.

T3 lesions: these tumors are almost always high grade, nodular, and very aggressive. Unfortunately, many may actually be under-staged tumors with the cancer already spread beyond the confines of the bladder. When an individual develops muscle invasive bladder cancer, major intervention is required to prevent spread and save the life of the individual.

T4 lesions: high grade invasive, aggressive tumors which have invaded adjacent organs. Many of these have also spread to distant parts of the body (are understaged) and are incurable.

WHAT ABOUT THE GRADE OF THE CANCER, HOW USEFUL IS IT IN PREDICTING PROGNOSIS?

Although not as predictive as stage, the cancer grade is an important prognostic indicator. The risk of progression for Grade 1 is 2%, Grade 2 is 11% and for Grade 3 is 45%.[4] As previously noted, the grade is clearly linked with the stage. Invasive tumors are almost all high grade.[5]

WHAT ELSE CAN BE USED TO PREDICT PROGRESSION?

A number of other factors may be utilized to help predict the likelihood of recurrence and progression of an individual's bladder cancer after treatment:[6]

---

[4] Heney NM, Ahmed S,Flanagan MJ, et al. Superficial bladder cancer: Progression and recurrence. J Urol1983;130:1083-1086.

[5] Torti FM, Lum BL, Aston D, et al. Superficial bladder cancer: The primacy grade in the development of invasive disease. J Clin Oncol 1987; 5:125-130.

[6] Ehab A. El-Gabry, M.D., Stephen E Strup, M.D., Leonard G. Gomella, M.D. AUA Update Series. Lesson 19, Volume 19: Superficial Bladder Cancer Epidemiology, Diagnosis, and Natural History Part 1: 150-151.

Tumor size: There generally is little difference in the recurrence rates of small tumors (tumors approximately 1-3 cm in size or ½-1 ½ inches in size). As tumors grow to mid size and larger, it is generally believed that recurrence rates are increased.

Tumor Configuration: More important than the size alone is the actual appearance of the tumor. Tumors that are papillary in appearance usually have a better prognosis than tumors that are solid (sessile or nodular).

Multifocality: When multiple tumors are present, scattered over various sites, the prognosis is worsened. If CIS is present in conjunction with bladder tumors, the rate of recurrence and progression is markedly worsened. Having multiple sites affected represents a widespread abnormal urothelium with an increased risk of future disease.

Abnormal DNA: The amount of abnormal DNA content in a cell can be analyzed. Higher grade tumors generally have an increased amount of abnormal DNA and have a higher recurrence and progression rate. The percentage of cells actively creating new DNA can also be measured. When this is increased, prognosis is worsened. These tests are often used to analyze abnormal cytology specimens.

p53: This gene is responsible for the production of a protein that is key in cell replication. An abnormal p53 gene can be detected and if present, increases the rate of cancer progression significantly.

Failure to respond to bladder treatment: As you will soon learn, there are a number of treatment options available to reduce the recurrence rate of bladder cancer (see Chapter Nine). Treatment failure itself is a negative prognostic indicator.

CHAPTER EIGHT
INITIAL SURGICAL TREATMENT
FOR BLADDER CANCER

An individual may be first diagnosed with bladder cancer when it is seen on X ray or ultrasound exam or found during a diagnostic cystoscopy. In this chapter, we will review how bladder tumors are removed from the body. Fortunately, urologists have instruments that can remove tumors without open surgery.

I'M SCHEDULED FOR A TURBT (TRANSURETHRAL RESECTION BLADDER TUMOR) AND BIOPSIES. CAN YOU EXPLAIN WHAT WILL OCCUR PRIOR TO THE OPERATION?

Your procedure will likely be scheduled at the hospital surgicenter as an outpatient. Depending on the extent of surgery and your general health, you may be required to stay in the hospital afterwards. There will be numerous forms to fill out, including consents for surgery and anesthesia. You will be asked whether or not you have a living will or power of attorney (see Chapter 15). Both the expected surgery and anesthesia planned will be fully discussed with you, including potential risks and alternatives. Your urologist will perform a history and physical exam to make sure you are fit for surgery. If you have multiple potentially serious medical problems, you probably have already had a pre operative visit with your internist, cardiologist or appropriate primary care physician. You will be asked whether or not you have any drug allergies, artificial joints, or other medical devices implanted, such as a pacemaker. An IV (intravenous line) will be inserted into a vein in your hand or arm. You will be wheeled on your stretcher to the cystoscopy room and then positioned on the cystoscopy table. Small paste on leads will be placed to monitor your heart and a small device will be clipped over your finger to monitor the level of oxygen in your blood. You will then be given your appropriate level of anesthesia. Depending on the size and location of the tumor(s) and the difficulty of the procedure, your urologist will likely make a recommendation to you regarding the level of anesthesia required. He may give more than one choice. Risks of each will be reviewed with you by the anesthesiologist or nurse anesthetist (a nurse specialized in giving anesthesia).

Your procedure may be done under:

Local with sedation: a numbing gel is squirted into your urethra and you are given intravenous sedation. Advantages include the lowest level of anesthesia, potentially with the least side effects and risks and quickest post op recovery from anesthesia. Many individuals are concerned they will experience pain. For small tumors and relatively minor surgery, this is an excellent form of anesthesia with very few patients experiencing pain or adverse reactions. If you do experience significant discomfort, your level of anesthesia can be changed to spinal or general.

Spinal anesthesia: accomplished by passing a fine needle into the lower spinal canal and injecting an anesthetic. Advantages include the ability to provide almost complete blockage of all pain and sensation during the surgery. The patient can continue to breathe on his own (a possible advantage for those with lung disease). Disadvantages include the occasional difficulty in giving the spinal (usually done rapidly with minimal pain, but sometimes difficult with pain), slower recovery from anesthesia (the length of spinal anesthetic is based on the amount and type of agent used and can generally be timed to match fairly closely the anticipated length of your procedure) and the possibility of a post spinal headache (not very common, but can last a day or more and be moderate to severe).

General anesthesia: delivered through IV medications and anesthesia in a gaseous mixture via a mask or endotracheal tube (a tube inserted down your throat into your trachea, your main airway). The choice of mask or endotracheal tube is generally decided by the anesthetist. This decision is based on the length of the anticipated procedure, your general health, and how easy it is to "ventilate" or provide oxygen to you with a mask alone. The advantage of general anesthesia is total blockade of all pain and sensation (you are unconscious). For healthy individuals with large tumors or with expected difficult surgery, this method is often the best form of anesthesia. For those in whom spinal anesthesia is not possible and a large tumor is present, general anesthesia is the best option.

YEARS AGO WHEN I HAD A MINOR SURGERY, I WAS REQUIRED TO HAVE A CHEST X RAY, EKG, AND MULTIPLE VIALS OF BLOOD FOR TESTING. FOR THIS SURGERY, I WAS TOLD NO TESTING IS REQUIRED. IS THIS CORRECT?

For many years, hospitals required indiscriminate preoperative testing, often including numerous lab studies, chest X ray and EKG. Today, the medical industry is more cost sensitive. Most centers will require only necessary tests based on your age, medical history, and medications. An EKG is often requested for those with heart disease and for individuals over the age of 50. Specific labs are required if you have a chronic illness or are taking medication which can change the bodies normal chemical balance. Reserving blood from the blood bank is rarely required unless you present with a low blood count from hematuria or from another illness.

HOW DOES THE UROLOGIST REMOVE THE BLADDER CANCER?

The urologist will often start by introducing a rigid cystoscope to examine the urethra and bladder. During the exam, your bladder will be filled with sterile water which travels through the scope. This is necessary to expand the bladder lumen fully, allowing a complete examination. Patients often are concerned too much fluid will be instilled, resulting in possible injury to the bladder or worse, a rupture. Because the water is instilled with only minimal pressure, bladder injury should not be a concern. The urologist can shut off the irrigation readily when the bladder is full and can empty the bladder at any time. After the cystoscopy is completed, the urologist then removes the bladder tumor(s).

If the tumors are small, he may simply use a biopsy forceps through the cystoscope (an instrument which has a small cup like end to remove pieces of tissue). Deep biopsies at the base of the tumor (especially when one is dealing with solid tumors as opposed to papillary variety) may be obtained using the same biopsy forceps. The tumors and deep biopsies are sent to the pathologist for examination. Additional biopsies from any suspicious areas or possibly the prostatic urethra may be done. After the tumor removal and biopsies are completed, electric current is used to stop any bleeding. The urologist steps on a pedal to turn the electric current on when the cable is touching the bleeding blood vessel.

For larger tumors, a resectoscope is required. Similar to a cystoscope, it is made of metal and is rigid. It is often larger than a cystoscope and has a special resection loop attached to remove tumors. Because they are larger, it may be necessary to first dilate the urethra to allow the resectoscope to be passed readily into the bladder. Dilation is done with smooth metal sounds which come in graduated sizes. The urologist starts with a small sound and gradually increases the size to stretch the urethra. Resectoscopes provide the capacity for continuous flow irrigation during the procedure. Sterile water runs into the bladder via the resectoscope through one port with excess fluid drained via a different port, allowing the urologist excellent visibility and speeding the surgery. The urologist begins his resection by first removing the tumor edge that is facing the inside of the bladder. The tumor is gradually resected down to the base. Usually, a deep resection is then accomplished through the base, into the deeper layer of bladder muscle. The resectoscope loop can be electrified to cauterize any bleeding points to stop bleeding.

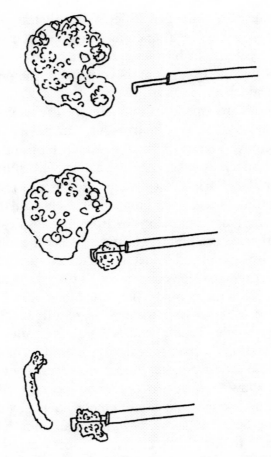

TRANSURETHRAL RESECTION BLADDER TUMOR (TURBT)

After fully completing the resection, the urologist will often do a bi-manual exam while the patient is under anesthesia. He does this by placing the gloved index finger into the rectum of the male patient, palpating upwards while simultaneously pressing down on the lower abdomen with his other hand. In the female, the opposing palpating hand is placed in the vaginal canal. After resecting a bladder tumor, a mass still palpable in the bladder wall would indicate residual, often serious bladder cancer. In addition to the presence of a mass on bimanual exam, the urologist will also check to see if the mass is mobile or fixed in position. A fixed mass would generally indicate spread of the tumor beyond the bladder with invasion into surrounding tissue, a very worrisome finding.

I WAS TOLD I WILL NEED A CATHETER AFTER MY TURBT. WHAT IS ITS PURPOSE, HOW UNCOMFORTABLE WILL IT BE, AND HOW LONG WILL I NEED IT?

A catheter is a plastic or rubber tube which is placed through the urethra into the bladder. It is kept in place by a fluid filled balloon, at the end of the catheter, which is inflated in the bladder. The tube allows for drainage of urine which may be mixed with blood after a TURBT. When small tumors are removed, a catheter is not usually required unless there is a concern that you may have difficulty urinating after the procedure because of an enlarged prostate, weak bladder or swelling of the urethra after instrumentation. After large tumors are resected, a catheter is often required. It serves the following purposes:

It allows one to monitor the amount of bleeding after surgery (although the urologist attempts to stop all bleeding, this is not always possible and bleeding may persist).

It provides for bladder irrigation if required. If much bleeding is present after surgery, it is important to avoid the possibility of blood clots forming and blocking the flow of urine. Irrigation can be done intermittently with a syringe or continuously via a 3 way catheter, which has a port for inflow and outflow of irrigant.

It keeps the bladder decompressed, which may be important if the resection was deep and bladder integrity is in question. The bladder may have been thinned markedly in the area of resection or biopsies. Decompression provides for reduced risk of leakage through the wall of the thinned bladder.

HOW UNCOMFORTABLE IS THE CATHETER?

Most individuals complain of some discomfort from their catheter. The most common complaint is a feeling of pressure in the bladder, often thought to be secondary to stimulating the bladder and resulting in a "bladder spasm". This sensation can often be reduced markedly with medication to relax the bladder. Sometimes pain medication is also required. The catheter may also cause irritation at the opening of the urethra, which can be reduced by being sure the catheter is kept clean at this site via gently cleansing and possibly applying an antibiotic ointment to the urethral opening.

HOW LONG DOES THE CATHETER NEED TO STAY IN?

If it was placed for bleeding, generally when the bleeding slows or stops over a day or two, the catheter will be removed. If it is in for a compromised bladder wall, it may need to remain for a week or more. When the catheter is removed, the urologist simply empties the balloon that holds it in place, and then gently pulls out the catheter. There is minimal discomfort during removal and generally a smile follows once it is out.

CAN ALL BLADDER TUMORS BE REACHED WITH A RESECTOSCOPE?

On occasion, a urologist may face an individual with a bladder tumor that cannot be reached. This is usually much more of an issue with male patients since the scope is required to pass through a much longer urethra to begin with, therefore reducing the amount of instrument available to work within the bladder. Contributing factors include:

Tumor location: tumors located at the dome (the very top part of the bladder or those just inside the bladder neck) may be extremely difficult to remove.

Body size: individuals who are markedly obese have distorted internal anatomy. Instruments may not be long enough to reach all bladder tumors.

Enlarged bladders: individuals with abnormally large bladders may have tumors beyond the reach of the resectoscope.

Bladder diverticulum: some bladders have an abnormal cavity called a diverticulum. If the opening to the diverticulum is small or if the diverticulum is large, bladder tumor removal may be difficult. In addition, the walls of the diverticulum are quite thin, making tumor removal more hazardous, as perforation is more likely to occur.

WHAT CAN MY UROLOGIST DO TO ENHANCE HIS ABILITY TO REMOVE TUMORS IN DIFFICULT LOCATIONS?

The experienced urologist uses several techniques to improve his chances of removing tumors that are difficult to reach. He will often keep the bladder under filled. Although this may reduce visibility, it will allow the tumor to be closer to the resectoscope. Another technique is to place manual pressure on the bladder from above. This is done by an assistant or by the urologist himself. By pushing down from above, tumors at the dome are displaced downwards. An additional technique, for the male patient, is operating through a perineal urethrostomy. The urologist makes a surgical opening into the urethra between the scrotum and rectum, allowing the resectoscope to move further into the bladder, bypassing much of the urethra.

Another option would be to use a laser. Laser fibers are flexible and may be able to reach a difficult tumor. The tumor may be effectively destroyed with laser energy; a disadvantage is no specimen is obtained.

Photodynamic therapy may afford additional results. With this novel technique, a chemical is instilled into the bladder, sensitizing the cancer cells to light energy. The entire bladder is then illuminated with laser light via a cystoscope. This treatment is not widely available at the present time and it is most effective for small tumors.

WHAT ARE THE COMPLICATIONS OF TURBT?

There are potential risks and complications of any surgical technique. Bladder tumor removal via resectoscope is usually safe and complication free. However, potential problems may arise:

Bleeding is usually present, but rarely severe. Some tumors are more vascular than others and will bleed more. In addition, the resection will involve the bladder wall and vascularity varies here as well. Transfusions are not generally required unless an individual starts with a low blood count from previous bleeding or medical condition. Bleeding can be an on going concern until the bladder completely heals weeks later. Catheterization and irrigation may be required. Just a small amount of blood will change the color of urine red. Urine that is punch colored or the color of rosé wine generally is not serious and will clear on its own. When the urine has large amounts of blood in it, the appearance generally looks like tomato juice, indicating serious bleeding requiring medical attention.

Bladder perforation may occur, especially with large tumors or those located on the lateral bladder walls. During resection of tumors on the lateral walls, the obturator nerve, which runs alongside the outside of the lateral bladder wall, may cause a strong muscle contraction. This contraction can abruptly move the bladder during a resection, resulting in a perforation. During resection of a large tumor with solid base, the urologist proceeds with deep resection of the tumor to remove the entire tumor and also determine whether or not it is a high stage tumor with muscle invasion. Bladder walls differ in size and integrity, and sometimes a perforation may occur. In addition, bladders which have previously been subject to some form of stress such as radiation or chemotherapy may have extremely poor integrity and are subject to pulling apart during a resection, resulting in a perforation. Bladder perforation is usually detected during the resection when the urologist sees fat (perivesical fat is located on the outside of the bladder). Sometimes, during a particularly bloody resection, the perforation may not be visible intraoperatively, but discovered when the lower abdomen becomes firm and distended (indicating that a large volume of fluid has passed into the abdomen). Small perforations are usually handled by stopping the procedure and maintaining a catheter for a week or more. Large perforations, especially those that communicate with the peritoneal cavity (the cavity that encases the bowels) generally require open surgical repair. Perforations can potentially spread cancer beyond the bladder.

Ureteral injury may occur when a tumor covers the ureter in the bladder. The ureter may be obscured by a bladder tumor, and the urologist may inadvertently resect it along with the tumor. In general, cutting current to remove a bladder tumor does not usually lead to long lasting problems as compared to cauterization, which is more likely to cause permanent blockage or obstruction of the ureter. If the urologist is working in the area of the ureter, he should avoid cauterization as much as possible. He may ask the anesthetist to inject an intravenous coloring agent which will turn the urine blue and allow visualization of the ureter. If he knows a ureter may be in jeopardy, he may insert a stent (a small plastic tube that traverses the ureter) for several weeks to allow the ureter to heal in an open fashion.

Urethral injury is infrequent and is almost always in males. A stricture or narrowed area of the urethra may result from irritation or injury from the resectoscope pressing on the urethra. Individuals that develop strictures complain of difficulty urinating, experiencing a slow or split stream. Strictures are usually readily handled with a number of urologic procedures.

Bladder tumor "seeding" may occur during the procedure. As the tumors are resected, cancer cells are released into the irrigant which fills the bladder. These cells may implant in other areas of the bladder traumatized during the procedure. It should be understood that the bladder is generally filled with urine, and tumor cells can naturally implant at other locations even without surgery. Implantation can be lessened during surgery by avoiding injury to other bladder areas and by the use of adjuvant intravesical chemotherapy. There have been numerous studies over the past decade showing a number of chemotherapy agents can be effective in decreasing initial tumor recurrence, possibly by preventing seeding. Reduction in recurrence may however be short lived. Previously, it was common practice to obtain multiple random bladder biopsies at the time of initial tumor resection. This was recommended to rule out the possibility of hidden CIS. Understanding these biopsy sites may increase the possibilities of tumor recurrence by tumor seeding, biopsies are now often limited to areas adjacent to the tumors removed and suspicious appearing areas only. CIS can be ruled out by using cytology, or by obtaining biopsies during future cystoscopy after the tumor has already been removed. When dealing with low grade tumors, random biopsies of the bladder will rarely show cancer.[1]

---

[1] van der Meijden A, Oosterlinck W, Brausi M, et al. Significance of bladder biopsies in Ta, T1 bladder tumors: a report from EORTC Genitourinary Tract Cancer Cooperative Group. EORTC-GU Group Superfical Bladder Committee EUR Urol. 1999; 35 (4): 267-271.

WHAT CAN I EXPECT AFTER MY TURBT IS FINISHED?

After your procedure, depending on the level of anesthesia and the extent of surgery, you will be brought either to the recovery room or back to the area where you were first prepared for your procedure. You will be released to home only when you have fully recovered from you anesthetic and are doing well.

NOW THAT MY BLADDER TUMOR HAS BEEN SUCCESS-FULLY REMOVED, MY UROLOGIST INFORMED ME I WILL NEED TO HAVE ANOTHER CYSTOSCOPY IN 3 MONTHS, IS THIS REALLY NECESSARY?

The recurrence rate for superficial bladder cancer can be as high as 60-90%. Recurrences can cause bleeding and other difficulties and are best handled sooner rather than later. In addition, depending on the initial tumor grade and stage, progression to a more serious form of bladder cancer is an ongoing concern. Surveillance cystoscopy is therefore recommended. Cystoscopy is still the best means to check for recurrent disease. It is however, an invasive procedure and should be accomplished only as often as required. For solitary, low grade, non invasive disease, follow up cystoscopy can be accomplished with the flexible cystoscope if available. If negative at three months, further cystoscopic exams can be done yearly and eventually lengthened even further. For those with multiple tumors, large tumors, high grade tumors or those who also have CIS, frequent cystoscopies, initially every three months are called for. As long as there are no recurrences, the time between cystoscopies can be lengthened. Cytology can also be utilized to reduce the number of cystoscopies. If recurrence or progression does occur, heightened scrutiny is again called for.

BESIDES A BLADDER TUMOR, MY CT SCAN INDICATED MY KIDNEY IS SWOLLEN BECAUSE OF A BLOCKAGE OF MY URETER. DID THE BLADDER TUMOR CAUSE THIS BLOCKAGE AND DOES IT MEAN MY PROGNOSIS IS WORSE?

There are many medical conditions that may result in hydroureteronephrosis (swelling of the kidney and ureter), having nothing to do with bladder cancer. It is also true large bladder tumors may grow into the wall of the bladder and cause ureteral obstruction at the level of the bladder. When this is found, the prognosis is usually poor, as the tumors involved are usually high grade and deeply invasive. On occasion, a superficial low grade tumor may grow directly into the ureteral opening. In this situation, prognosis is not generally any worse, as the blockage has not occurred from an invasive tumor.

DURING ROUTINE FOLLOW UP, I WAS FOUND TO HAVE BLADDER CANCER GROWING INTO MY PROSTATE. HOW SHOULD THIS BE TREATED?

The urologist will determine if the cancer is superficial or invasive (growing deeper than the subepithelial connective tissue or stroma). Superficial disease is generally amenable to transurethral resection and treatment with intravesical BCG (Chapter 9), while deeply invasive disease often warrants radical cystectomy.

MY UROLOGIST HAS RECOMMENDED AN IVP EVERY FEW YEARS TO RULE OUT DISEASE RECURRENCE IN THE UPPER TRACTS (KIDNEY, PELVIS, OR URETER). IS THIS WARRANTED?

A number of studies have shown individuals with high risk superficial disease should be closely monitored with yearly IVP or IVP after the development of a positive cytology. Those with high risk disease treated successfully with BCG are still at risk for upper tract disease and should be carefully monitored. For those with low risk disease, checking the upper tracts less frequently would be appropriate. Unfortunately, when upper tract disease develops, prognosis is markedly worsened, with many individuals eventually dying from their cancer.

IS IT EVER RECOMMENDED TO REMOVE THE BLADDER (RADICAL CYSTECTOMY) FOR SUPERFICIAL BLADDER CANCER?

When an individual has diffuse, high grade cancer of the bladder, even when superficial, bladder removal may be warranted. Many may have widespread carcinoma in situ (CIS) in conjunction with papillary disease. One can expect a high rate of recurrence and a high rate of progression to invasive disease. Generally, intravesical therapy is tried first. If this therapy is unsuccessful, repeated therapy or alternate intravesical therapies can be tried. However, with failure of intravesical therapy, further trials may prove to be equally ineffective and lead to unnecessary delay for potentially definitive curative therapy. Many recommend removal of the bladder if two courses of six weeks of BCG are ineffective. Therefore, radical cystectomy is a treatment option for any individual who is thought to be at significant risk for progression to muscle invasive and potentially metastatic disease.

IS THERE ANY ROLE FOR RADIATION THERAPY FOR THE TREATMENT OF SUPERFICIAL BLADDER CANCER?

For individuals with recurrent disease despite tumor removal and intravesical therapy (see Chapter Nine), progression to a more serious, muscle invasive disease is common. The patient at high risk for progression must consider radical cystectomy. If the individual is not a candidate for radical cystectomy because of poor health or the individual refuses cystectomy, radiation therapy can be considered. There are no good studies available and it is difficult to assess the efficacy of radiation alone since it is always combined with TURBT and the completeness of tumor resection is an uncertain variable. In general, radiation plays a minimal role in the treatment of superficial bladder cancer.

CHAPTER NINE
INTRAVESICAL THERAPY

For those individuals whose bladder tumors are at high risk for recurrence or progression, instillation of agents directly into the bladder can be worthwhile. The forms of therapeutic agents come in two groups: chemotherapy or immunotherapy. It is fortunate the bladder is readily accessible to these agents, allowing for direct action with minimal systemic side effects.

WHICH PATIENTS SHOULD HAVE INTRAVESICAL THERAPY?

Those individuals at high risk for recurrence and or progression should be considered for this therapy. Individuals with multiple or diffuse superficial tumors, large tumors, high grade tumors, superficially invasive tumors, those with recurrence within one year, or individuals with CIS all should be considered for this treatment. In addition, those with positive cytology after resection or patients with persistent superficial tumors which could not be removed should also be considered.

HOW IS THE INTRAVESICAL AGENT PUT INTO THE BLADDER?

The agent is passed via a catheter into the bladder. The passage of the catheter generally takes just a few seconds in a woman, and perhaps ten seconds in a man. The urethral meatus (the outermost part of the urethra) is first cleansed with an antiseptic solution and then the catheter, which is made slippery with a sterile lubricant, is inserted up the urethra and into the bladder. On passage of the catheter, there is minor, short lived discomfort which may be reduced by an injection up the urethra with numbing medication. The various therapeutic agents are not painful during the infusion but may cause side effects afterwards. Depending on the agent instilled, the patient is asked not to void for a period of time afterwards to allow the agent to have its maximal effect on the bladder lining.

WHICH AGENT OR FORM OF THERAPY IS MOST EFFECTIVE?

Careful trials have confirmed that immunotherapy with Bacillus Calmette-Guerin (BCG) is the most effective form of intravesical therapy presently available.

MY UROLOGIST TELLS ME THAT BCG IS A BACTERIUM. ISN'T THIS DANGEROUS TO INFUSE INTO THE BLADDER?

BCG is a living but attenuated form of tuberculosis bacteria. Similar to other living vaccines, it is used to create a heightened immunity. There are a number of precautions which must be taken to make sure the BCG is infused safely. BCG should not be infused immediately or shortly after tumor resection. Several weeks should be allowed to pass so the BCG does not gain access into open blood vessels. In addition, BCG should not be infused if the individual has a urinary infection, has active bleeding, or if the catheterization is traumatic and causes bleeding. It should not be used in patients whose immune system is seriously compromised or for those on steroids, which can decrease the immune system.

HOW DOES BCG WORK?

The exact mechanism(s) of BCG is still not fully understood. It is known BCG actually attaches to and enters cancer cells. BCG is thought to trigger an increased immune reaction in the bladder, thereby killing off cancer cells.

WHAT PRECAUTIONS MUST BE TAKEN AFTER I RECEIVE BCG?

BCG is held in the bladder for two hours. One should not hold it longer as adverse reactions are increased. The individual should then void into a toilet at home, preferably in a seated position to avoid splashing. After voiding, the toilet is disinfected with bleach. Since BCG can be shed from the urethra after treatment for several days, condoms should be used or one should abstain from sexual relations for at least 48 hours after treatment.

HOW EFFECTIVE IS BCG?

Studies have shown an approximately 40% reduction in tumor recurrence in those treated with BCG as compared with those without treatment.[1] For those with CIS, the reduction is even greater at approximately 70%.[2] For individuals with residual tumors after resection, complete response is generally about 60%.[3] Despite intravesical therapy, ultimately between 10-20% of individuals with superficial bladder cancer will develop muscle invasive disease.

WHAT TYPE OF TREATMENT REGIMEN IS RECOMMENDED?

After a 6 week induction course of weekly BCG, treatment is often repeated with 3 weekly treatments at 3 months, 6 months and then every 6 months for up to 3 years. This regimen was shown to decrease recurrences and increase complete responses as compared to induction treatment alone. Unfortunately, despite initial success, over long periods of time, many will experience disease recurrence and progression.[4] Treatment regimens can be individualized based on the patient's progress and his adverse reactions to treatment, which generally increase with repeated cycles.

---

[1] Lamm DL: Long term results of intravesical therapy for superficial bladder cancer. Urol Clin North Am 1992; 19: 573-580.

[2] Lamm DL: Carcinoma in situ: Urol Clin North Am 1992; 19: 499-508.

[3] Bosman SA: BCG in the management of superficial bladder cancer. Urol 1984;23: 82-87.

[4] Lamm DL, Blumenstein BA, Crissman JD, et al. Maintenance bacillus Calmette-Guerin immunotherapy for recurrent TA, T1, and carcinoma in situ transitional cell carcinoma of the bladder: a randomized Southwest Oncology Group Study. J Urol. 2000; 163 (4): 1124-1129.

WHAT ARE THE ADVERSE REACTIONS?

Adverse reactions are side effects of treatment. Approximately 95% of individuals will tolerate treatments well. Adverse reactions may be mild. Common reactions include cystitis (inflammation of the bladder characterized by burning on urination), hematuria, mild fever, malaise, and nausea. These symptoms generally pass without any treatment. For bothersome symptoms, various medications may prove helpful. Your physician can prescribe medication for burning or urinary frequency. For those with persistent cystitis, antibiotics can be utilized. For individuals experiencing severe symptoms lasting more than 48 hours, isoniazid, an anti-tuberculous drug can be prescribed. A short course of 3 days, starting the day before the next dose of BCG can be used to prevent severe side effects. Fortunately severe reactions resulting in sepsis, a life threatening condition characterized by high fever, chills and drop in blood pressure, is exceedingly rare. Sepsis would be treated in a hospital with triple anti-tuberculous drugs, steroids, and broad spectrum antibiotics. There are other serious adverse reactions which may require dose reduction or discontinuation. These are all rare and include: inflammation of the prostate, persistent hematuria, hepatitis, inflammation of the testicles and or epididymis, bladder contraction, ureteral obstruction, joint pain or inflammation of the lungs.

CAN ADVERSE REACTIONS BE REDUCED?

As treatment cycles progress, generally adverse reactions increase in severity, the most common being cystitis. Patients should not receive additional doses until they are asymptomatic. Studies have demonstrated increasing the intervals between treatments and reducing the dose of the BCG can still result in perhaps equal efficacy, but with reduced toxicity.

WHY DOES MY UROLOGIST WAIT SIX WEEKS AFTER BCG TO REPEAT CYSTOSCOPY, TO SEE IF IT HAS BEEN EFFECTIVE?

BCG therapy results in marked inflammation of the bladder wall. Cystoscopy done too soon after therapy would reveal a markedly reddened surface, making finding a bladder tumor difficult. Furthermore, microscopically, there will be severe reactive changes, complicating the pathologist's job, as deciding between changes from the BCG and recurrent cancer, would be extremely difficult.

WHAT HAPPENS IF MY BLADDER CANCER COMES BACK AFTER BCG?

Recurrence of bladder cancer after the initial induction course, or relapse after complete response, would indicate failure of therapy. When two or more courses result in recurrence or when recurrence develops during the first six to twelve months after induction and maintenance therapy, patients generally are felt to have disease which is at higher risk for progression. A high percentage of patients who are complete responders remain tumor free for up to five years. However, with the passage of more time, additional patients will have late recurrences. For those with late recurrences (two to three years after therapy), most will respond to repeat BCG therapy.

WHAT OTHER FORMS OF INTRAVESICAL IMMUNOTHER-APY ARE THERE?

Interferon (alpha 2b, Intron A) is recognized as potentially beneficial for bladder cancer treatment despite the lack of FDA approval at this time. Interferon is naturally produced by the immune system and has antitumor effects.

HOW EFFECTIVE IS INTERFERON?

Interferon is not as effective as BCG. Complete response for bladder cancer and CIS is generally lower than with BCG. Response is dose related with better results when a 50 million to 100 million unit dose is given. Interferon is generally used as second line therapy for those who have failed BCG or cannot tolerate BCG therapy.

WHAT ARE THE SIDE EFFECTS OF INTERFERON THERAPY?

Intravesical interferon is generally well tolerated. A low grade fever and flu like symptoms occur in less than 30% of patients. Side effects do not increase with higher doses.

MY UROLOGIST HAS RECOMMENDED COMBINATION THERAPY WITH BCG AND INTERFERON AFTER I FAILED BCG THERAPY. IS THIS ACCEPTABLE?

Recent studies have shown the combination of BCG with Interferon results in greater efficacy in treating bladder cancer than either agent alone.[5] A lower dose of BCG is mixed with Interferon and both are infused via a catheter into the bladder. Since a lower dose of BCG is used, the treatments are generally well tolerated. After an induction phase of 6 treatments, the patient is cystoscoped to determine response. If there is a good response, maintenance therapy with repeated treatments follow.

WHAT ABOUT INTRAVESICAL CHEMOTHERAPY?

The agents which are most commonly used are Mitomycin, Thiotepa, Valrubicin, and Doxorubicin. Many studies have shown a reduction in recurrence rates with immediate post tumor resection use of Mitomycin and Thiotepa. By giving single dose therapy, toxicity is limited. However, long term recurrence rates are just as high in

---

[5]   O'Donnell MA, Krohn J, DeWolf WC. Salvage intravesical therapy with interferon alpha 2b plus low dose bacillus Calmette-Guerin is effective in patients with superficial bladder cancer in whom bacillus Calmette-Guerin alone previously failed. J Urol. 2001; 166: 1300-1305.

the treated patients as compared with the untreated. A recent study reviewed prior studies comparing the use of BCG versus Mitomycin C in reducing recurrence and progression in those at high risk. Tumor recurrence was significantly lower with intravesical BCG than with Mitomycin C. However, there was no difference in progression of disease.[6] Consequently, intravesical chemotherapy is generally used in those individuals who have failed intravesical immunotherapy or who are not candidates for immunotherapy.

ARE THERE ANY OTHER OPTIONS FOR TREATMENT OF RECURRENT SUPERFICIAL BLADDER CANCER?

Laser therapy can be used to destroy superficial bladder cancers. It can prove particularly useful for treatment of tumors that cannot be reached with a standard resectoscope (such as tumors on the dome of the bladder in an obese individual). Generally, it is well tolerated with minimal bleeding. The disadvantage is the lack of pathologic specimen.

Another modality, photodynamic therapy, was first reported in 1976. A photosensitizer is injected intravenously followed by whole bladder laser light therapy. Photofrin is approved by the FDA as a photosensitizer. It accumulates at a higher rate in rapidly dividing cells (the norm for cancer). When activated by light energy, the photosensitizer causes cell destruction. This therapy can eradicate superficial disease and CIS refractory to BCG therapy. Unfortunately, the therapy causes severe local inflammation and can lead to bladder contracture (shrunken bladder) in up to 20% of patients. It is accomplished under general anesthesia. Also, because the skin is also sensitized, the individual having treatment needs to avoid sun light or bright light for approximately 6 weeks. This therapy is available in only limited tertiary care centers. It may be justified as

---

[6]   Shelley MD, Wilt TJ, et al. Intravescial Bacillus Calmette-Guerin Is Superior to Mitomycin C in Reducing Tumour Recurrence in High-Risk Superficial Bladder Cancer: A Meta-Analysis of Randomized Trials. BJU Int 2004; 93: 485-490.

a last option in the hopes of avoiding cystectomy. Initial response rates may be as high as 50%.[7]

WHAT ELSE CAN I DO TO HELP PREVENT WORSENING BLADDER CANCER?

If you are still smoking, quit! Studies have shown those patients with bladder cancer that continue to smoke do worse than those who quit. Likewise, avoid exposure to any toxins which can lead to bladder cancer. Additionally, megadoses of vitamins in conjunction with BCG have been shown to reduce recurrence rates by as much as 40%, primarily in low grade, superficial disease.[8] Antioxidant vitamins in combination were used.

---

[7]   Shackley DC, Briggs C, Gilhooley A, et al. Photodynamic therapy for superficial bladder cancer under local anesthetic. BJU Int.2002; 89:665-670.

[8]   Lamm DL,RiggsDR, Shriver JS, et al. Megadose vitamins in bladder cancer: a double blind clinical trial. J Urol 1994; 151(1): 21-26.

CHAPTER TEN
INVASIVE BLADDER CANCER

In this chapter, we review the presentation, workup, and therapies for invasive bladder cancer. Invasive bladder cancer represents a subset of bladder cancer that grow into the bladder muscle. Approximately 20-30% of all bladder cancers are invasive. These cancers are aggressive and grow outside the bladder into surrounding tissues and organs, or spread (metastasize) into the lymph system or into the blood vessels. Invasive bladder cancers are life threatening and require an aggressive approach.

HOW DO INVASIVE BLADDER CANCERS PRESENT?

They present in an identical fashion as superficial bladder cancers. They may present with hematuria, irritative voiding symptoms, or can be found by accident on an ultrasound or X ray exam. On occasion, an individual may pass pieces of the tumor in his urine.

DO INVASIVE BLADDER CANCERS ALWAYS FORM AFTER A RECURRENCE AND PROGRESSION OF SUPERFICIAL BLADDER CANCER?

The vast majority do follow an initial presentation with superficial disease. However, approximately 25% of patients first present with serious invasive bladder cancer.

ARE INVASIVE BLADDER CANCERS GENERALLY HIGH GRADE AS WELL?

Invasive bladder cancers are almost always high grade. They are aggressive cancers and can spread rapidly. They are usually larger than superficial bladder cancers.

HOW DO INVASIVE BLADDER CANCERS SPREAD?

These cancers can spread directly through the bladder wall, invading tissues outside the bladder and adjacent organs such as the prostate. They can spread via lymphatics, first to the pelvic lymph nodes and then throughout the body through the lymphatic system. More rapid spread to distant organs can occur through the venous system.

ONCE THE CANCER HAS SPREAD THROUGH THE BLADDER WALL, IS CURE STILL POSSIBLE?

Radical cystectomy will cure approximately 75% of patients whose cancer is confined to the bladder muscle. Although individuals with minimal spread of cancer beyond the bladder may at times be cured with surgical removal of the bladder, even minimal disease outside the bladder may also be accompanied by metastatic disease, which cannot be cured by surgery alone. Therefore, microscopic spread through the bladder wall is a very bad prognostic finding. In general, larger cancers which have spread beyond the bladder to contiguous areas have a worse prognosis than cancers confined to the bladder with early spread to the surrounding lymph nodes. The more nodes involved outside the bladder by cancer, the worse the prognosis.

HOW IS INVASIVE BLADDER CANCER STAGED?

Invasive bladder cancer is often recognizable to the urologist by its appearance during cystoscopy. These cancers are generally large, sometimes multi-focal, and solid in appearance as compared to the fine papillary appearance of superficial bladder cancers. During the transurethral resection of the tumor, the urologist can generally tell the tumor is invading into the deeper portions of the bladder wall.

The pathologist's report will then indicate the grade of the cancer and the depth of invasion. If the tumor invades into muscle, it is an invasive tumor. Further staging would then include a CT Scan or MRI to assess local contiguous spread, lymph node spread, or more distant spread of the cancer. A chest X ray is also routine. If there are any suspicious areas, a CT Scan of the chest is ordered. A bone scan is generally not required unless the individual has had a new onset of bony pain that is not explained by injury or arthritis.

IS THE INITIAL TREATMENT OF INVASIVE BLADDER CANCER ANY DIFFERENT THAN TREATMENT FOR SUPERFICIAL BLADDER CANCER?

In both cases, the first step is a cystoscopy and removal of the tumor. For smaller superficial tumors, removal can sometimes be accomplished with biopsy forceps alone. For larger tumors, a resectoscope is used. In the case of a large invasive cancer which clearly is growing deep into the bladder, the urologist may choose not to remove the entire tumor since further surgery will be required and there is little to be gained by resecting more (and possibly more to be lost with a greater chance of serious bleeding or a bladder perforation with a more extensive resection). If however, the individual will not be a candidate for open surgery (due to advanced age or other medical risk factors), a more thorough resection may be advisable to prevent recurrence of future hematuria, or perhaps to allow for an alternate form of therapy such as a "bladder sparing" regimen, consisting of transurethral resection, radiation, and chemotherapy.

WHY CAN'T JUST THE SECTION OF BLADDER WITH CANCER BE REMOVED SURGICALLY TO CURE ME?

In a small percentage of individuals a partial cystectomy, removing just part of the bladder, is possible, and may be the preferred form of open surgery. This procedure can generally be accomplished if the cancer is located in an accessible area of the bladder such as the dome, is not multi-focal, or too large. Many tumors are too large, are multi-focal, or are in an inaccessible area, and therefore are not treatable with partial cystectomy. Furthermore, even when an individual presents with a cancer which is treatable via partial cystectomy, removal of the entire bladder may be preferable since recurrent, invasive disease in the remaining bladder is probable. For the elderly or those in poor health, and others with a limited life expectancy, partial cystectomy may be ideal if doable.

HOW SUCCESSFUL IS RADICAL CYSTECTOMY?

If the cancer is still confined to the bladder, long term survival free of cancer is to be expected in approximately 75-80%. There are reports indicating possible cure in some individuals with minimal disease outside the bladder.

WHAT NEEDS TO BE DONE PRIOR TO RADICAL CYSTECTOMY?

Radical cystectomy is a major surgery with potential complications. You therefore, need to be in the best possible medical condition prior to surgery. Your health care history will be reviewed by your urologist. If you have specific medical conditions such as heart disease or respiratory disease, a referral to the specialist or primary care physician overseeing management of these conditions is usually warranted to make sure your risk factors have been corrected or improved, to allow for safe surgery. If you have a medical condition which places you at substantial risk of a major complication, it should be addressed prior to proceeding with a surgery of this extent. For example, if you have a heart condition, such as an irregular heart beat, medication may need to be adjusted. Some patients may need to go on lung medication to improve their lung function. On occasion, an individual may need to even have surgery for a blocked heart vessel prior to going ahead with a radical cystectomy. If you still are smoking, you should definitely stop at least two weeks prior to surgery.

You will need to discontinue any medications that can affect your ability to clot during surgery. These may include coumadin and aspirin and other medications which keep your blood from readily clotting. Some vitamins such as Vitamin E can also affect clotting and should be stopped. Herbal remedies will also need to be reviewed with your urologist, as some may affect your ability to clot. Your urologist will go over the medications and let you know which will need to be discontinued prior to surgery. If you drink more than the equivalent of 2 ounces of alcohol per day, it is important to stop drinking alcohol preferably at least a week or more prior to surgery. If you are an alcoholic and drink large quantities of alcohol on a regular basis, you will face the possibility of delirium tremens (DTs) after surgery when you cannot drink alcohol. DTs is a serious medical complication with a high mortality rate. If you have any doubts regarding your consumption of alcohol, you should discuss this with your urologist.

You may wish to donate blood which will be held in the blood bank for you exclusively during or after surgery. These units of blood are called autologous units and may be transfused only into you. Your urologist will advise you if it is necessary for you to donate blood. If you do choose to donate blood, generally a unit can be given every 7-10 days. It is advisable to take iron supplements during donation so your body can quickly rebuild its blood supply prior to surgery.

If you have experienced a recent illness which has weakened you, it is important to be fully recovered prior to proceeding with the operation. Illness may result in a state of malnutrition. If you have experienced recent weight loss, it may be important to take protein supplements to build up your body prior to surgery.

Because your urologist will be using a piece of your bowel to create a new urinary drainage system, your small and large bowel will need to be thoroughly cleaned out prior to surgery. Your urologist will prescribe cleansing agents such as Golytely or Fleet Phospho-soda the day before surgery to rid the bowel of fecal contents. It is also standard to take a number of antibiotic pills the day before surgery to reduce the bacterial count in the bowel. You will be on "clear liquids" the day before with nothing to eat or drink after midnight. Your urologist will give you detailed instructions regarding the bowel prep and a prescription for the antibiotics.

Getting a good night's sleep the evening before surgery will help you deal with the initial anxiety as you travel to the hospital. Ask your physician for a "sleeping pill" if you know you will be facing a sleepless night.

If you are very anxious about your upcoming surgery, talk to your urologist or primary care physician. A prescription for medication to reduce anxiety may be appropriate. For those individuals who wish to "go natural," various techniques such as meditation, guided imagery, or Reiki can be practiced prior to and after surgery to reduce stress and anxiety and enhance your recovery. (See Chapter 14) These modalities are generally available in most communities. If you need help in learning these techniques, ask your physician for a referral or call your hospital for resources in your community.

WHAT HAPPENS PRIOR TO GOING TO THE OPERATING ROOM?

An intravenous line will be inserted into your arm. In many hospitals, it is also routine to pass an epidural catheter into your lower back. The nurse and anesthesiologist will review your chart and ask you numerous questions. Your surgical consent will need to be signed, as well as consent for anesthesia. Your urologist will visit with you and may repeat a physical exam prior to proceeding. Either your urologist or an enterostomy nurse may mark your skin for the future site of your ostomy. The ostomy site should be away from any skin folds or scar tissue, preferably below your belt line and accessible to you for ostomy care.

WHAT STANDARD PREPARATIONS ARE TAKEN AT THE BEGINNING OF SURGERY FOR BLADDER REMOVAL?

While still awake, you will be transferred onto the operating room table and secured on it. If an epidural has not already been placed, one may be inserted. You may have an additional intravenous line placed. Next, your anesthesiologist will have you breathe through a mask placed over your nose and mouth. You will be given a mixture of agents which will allow you to become relaxed. Further anesthetics will result in an unconscious state. At this time, an endotracheal tube will be passed down your windpipe to provide oxygen, which is delivered automatically by a respirator, controlled by the anesthesiologist. The anesthesiologist will continuously monitor your heart rate, blood pressure, electrocardiogram, and tissue oxygenation throughout your operation. Fluid balance may also be measured via an intravenous line passed close to your heart. Urine output will be followed. Antibiotics will be infused intravenously. Usually, compression stockings will be secured around your legs. These stockings periodically squeeze the legs to prevent blood from becoming stagnant, lowering the risk of blood clots forming in your legs, which can occur when you lie completely motionless for extended periods of time. A nasogastric tube will be passed through your nostril down your esophagus into the stomach, draining the stomach secretions during and after the surgery. A grounding pad will be placed on your side to allow for the safe use of electric current which is used to sometimes cut tissue and often in the cauterization of small bleeding vessels to stop bleeding. Your abdomen will be prepared for surgery by shaving any hair and prepping the skin with an antiseptic solution. Female patients will have the vagina prepped with antiseptics as well. The surgical field will then be draped with sterile towels and sheets to prevent contamination from surrounding non-sterilized areas. Your upper body may be kept warm with a warming blanket. Your surgical nurse, surgeon, and assistant will all have thoroughly cleaned their hands and arms (scrubbed) and will then don a sterile gown and gloves. Their hair will be covered with a surgical cap, and they will be wearing masks over their mouths to prevent any contamination of the sterilized surgical field.

EXPLAIN THE BASICS OF SURGERY FOR BLADDER REMOVAL.

The standard operation is called Radical Cystectomy. This operation is accomplished through an incision which extends down the middle of the abdomen beginning at the level of the umbilicus and extending down to the pubic bone. The peritoneum (the sac around your intestines) is opened. The surgeon will examine the abdomen to make sure there is no evidence of cancer spread. Removal of the lymph nodes from the pelvis around the bladder is accomplished. The bladder is removed in its entirety along with the prostate and seminal vesicles in the male. In the female, the uterus and vagina are adjacent to the bladder and may be involved with local spread of cancer beyond the bladder. Consequently, the uterus and part of the vagina are removed. Since most females having a cystectomy are well past menopause, the ovaries are also removed, thus avoiding the possibility of future diseases including ovarian cancer.

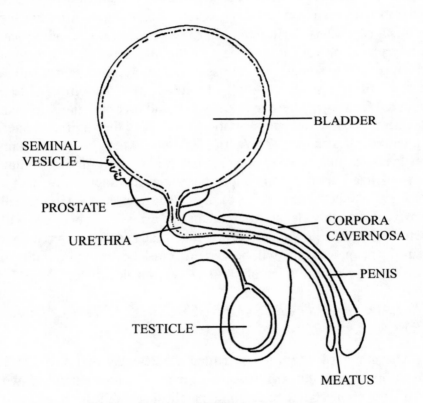

MALE GENITOURINARY SYSTEM

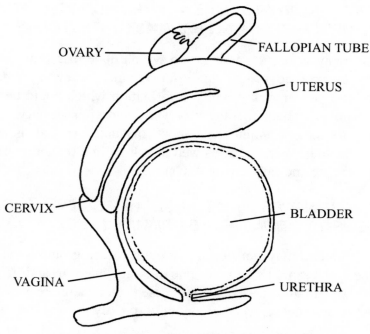

OVARY — FALLOPIAN TUBE

— UTERUS

CERVIX — BLADDER

VAGINA — URETHRA

FEMALE GENITOURINARY SYSTEM

Once the bladder and surrounding organs are removed, the urinary tract must be reconstructed. This is most often accomplished by sewing the ends of the ureters into a piece of ileum (a section of small intestine) which is brought out through the skin as an ostomy. This form of reconstruction is called an ileal loop diversion. Since this reconstruction involves the urinary tract, the ostomy is referred to as a urostomy. Prior to sewing the ureters into the ileum, a biopsy of the ends of both ureters is examined by a pathologist to make sure there is no carcinoma in situ present. If cancer is found at the end of the ureter, this section is removed and the next higher level is examined by the pathologist to assure the ureter is free of cancer at the implantation site. If a neobladder is being planned, the prostatic urethra is examined by the pathologist to assure no cancer is present prior to proceeding further. (See Chapter 11)

IS IT NECESSARY TO HAVE A LYMPH NODE DISSECTION ACCOMPLISHED DURING RADICAL CYSTECTOMY?

For many years, it was believed lymph node dissection served mainly to provide prognostic information. Knowing whether nodes have cancer was valuable information which could be used to determine if chemotherapy was warranted after surgery. More recently, a number of studies have shown that doing a nodal dissection may prove to be therapeutic as well, resulting in a reduction of risk for recurrence and improvement in survival.

WHY IS IT NECESSARY TO USE A PIECE OF BOWEL IN RECONSTRUCTION OF THE URINARY TRACT?

The ureters may not be long enough to bring out to the skin surface at the same location for one drainage bag. In addition, the ureters are small and easily compressed, and therefore would be subject to obstruction when brought out directly.

IS IT NECESSARY TO HAVE MY URETHRA REMOVED AT THE TIME OF RADICAL CYSTECTOMY?

Transitional cell cancer extending into the urethra of a female patient or the prostatic urethra of a male patient would generally require urethrectomy at the time of cystectomy. Urethrectomy requires more dissection, potential for bleeding and infection, and possibly increased post operative drainage. It should therefore be performed only when necessary. Cancer located close to the bladder neck may raise the odds of cancer developing in a urethra which is left behind. The status of the urethra can be followed post cystectomy with washings sent for cytology. If cancer subsequently develops, a urethrectomy can be accomplished as a separate operation long after cystectomy has been done.

WHAT IS THE TYPICAL POSTOPERATIVE COURSE?

At the conclusion of surgery, generally while still in the operating room, the endotracheal tube is removed when the patient is awake enough to breathe on his own. The patient will then be brought to the recovery room where he will be carefully observed by trained nurses in conjunction with the anesthesiologist and urologist. The individual is kept in the recovery room until conscious, breathing on his own and stable. Recovery room stays may be short, on the order of 30 minutes, or may extend to several hours, depending on how the individual is doing. If doing well, the patient will then be transferred to a floor in the hospital. If the individual's surgery was particularly complicated, extended, or if the individual is unstable (irregular heart beat, low blood pressure, inability to be taken off the respirator), or if the individual has significant medical problems or has experienced a complication from surgery, transfer to an ICU (intensive care unit) may be warranted. In the ICU, there exists a much higher ratio of nurses to patients than on a standard postoperative floor, allowing for constant surveillance and care for critical patients. Also, if a respirator is required postoperatively, initial treatment in an ICU is usually necessary.

After transfer to the floor from the recovery room, the patient is often kept on bed rest for the rest of the day. The nasogastric tube is left in and placed to gentle suction to remove excess stomach fluids. Initially, nothing is allowed by mouth other than ice chips or sips of water. Adequate fluids and some nutrition are given via an intravenous catheter. By the following day, patients are often out of bed and sometimes walking with assistance. Sequential stockings on the lower legs are removed while ambulating, and discontinued once the individual is able to move about well. Traditionally, nasogastric tubes have been left in until the bowel activity returns (generally 3-4 days). This is generally heralded by the passing of flatus (gas) or the presence of active bowel sounds, which will be checked by your urologist with a stethoscope. Recent studies have indicated nasogastric drainage for this length of time may not be necessary and may impede normal breathing, leading to other problems. Some urologists are therefore removing the tubes earlier. Feeding is gradually introduced however, once bowel activity has returned.

The patient will be encouraged to do deep breathing exercises to prevent lung collapse. This process is generally assisted with a small device called a spirometer. If the individual has a history of lung disease or is congested post-operatively, respiratory treatments with inhaled medication may be instituted and provided by a respiratory therapist.

Pain post-op is initially treated often via the epidural catheter. Intravenous medication may be given as an alternative and switched to oral pain meds once the individual is tolerating liquids. Many physicians order a PCA (patient controlled anesthesia) in which the patient pushes a button that releases pain medication via an intravenous line into the blood stream. Maximal amounts of drug administered are carefully controlled by settings on the PCA to allow safe, effective analgesia.

During the post-op period, you will meet regularly with an enterostomy nurse who will teach you the mechanics of caring for an ostomy and handling the ostomy appliance. Gradually, your pain will diminish, strength will increase, and diet will be advanced. Drains placed intraoperatively to siphon off any excess fluids from the abdomen will be removed when no longer needed.

Depending on the individual's age, general health, the surgery itself, and whether any complications have occurred, discharge to home can be expected after approximately seven to ten days.

WHAT ARE THE MOST FREQUENT OPERATIVE COMPLICATIONS AFTER RADICAL CYSTECTOMY?

For most patients in reasonably good health, few if any complications are the rule. A host of complications can occur with any major surgical procedure and hospital stay. The major complications associated with Radical Cystectomy include:

Intraoperative:

Bowel injury: During difficult dissection, small intestines may be inadvertently opened. These injuries are usually immediately recognized and repaired without difficulty. During removal of the bladder, the rectum may be entered. Assuming the patient has had a complete bowel prep prior to surgery, the rectum is usually readily repaired.

Vascular injury: During removal of the pelvic lymph nodes, entry into a major vein or artery may result in significant blood loss. Smaller, inconsequential veins or branches into larger veins are usually ligated with a suture or cauterized shut. Larger veins and arteries require repair with a fine vascular suture and needle. Troublesome bleeding can also occur during removal of the bladder and from deep in the pelvis after the bladder and prostate are removed. Bleeding is stopped through suture ligation, vascular clips, or cautery.

Post operative:

Abscess: An abscess is a pocket of pus located deep within the body. It may form from a bowel or urine leak, and generally will require drainage since antibiotics alone may not resolve it. If percutaneous drainage (drainage through the skin) is possible, the radiologist will drain the abscess. If this is not possible, the urologist will need to open the incision or make a new incision to allow the pus to be drained. A sizable abscess will generally not be cured without proper drainage. Left untreated, an abscess can result in sepsis, a life threatening bacterial infection.

Bowel leak: When the bowel is reconnected after removing the section for the urinary diversion, healing may not be adequate and bowel contents may leak into the abdomen. A bowel leak often will present as a failure of the bowel to return to normal function, resulting in a distended abdomen with poor bowel sounds. Distention, ileus (poor bowel function) may occur after the bowels are working well and feeding has been going on for some time. Evaluation is usually accomplished with CT Scan and oral contrast. Immediate surgical correction may be necessary. Left untreated, a bowel leak will generally lead to an abscess or possibly a fistula (a drainage tract from the bowel which may extend out through the incision or drain). The incidence of bowel leak is increased if bowel has been exposed to prior radiation, most often from radiation used to treat prostate cancer in men and uterine cancer in women.

Bowel obstruction: When a piece of bowel is separated from the intestine to create the new urinary drainage system, the remaining bowel must be reanastomosed (brought back together). This may be accomplished via sewing the bowel together or through the use of staples. Sometimes the opening of the bowel connection may be obstructed secondary to swelling. If an obstruction does not clear after a reasonable time, reoperation may be required.

Erectile dysfunction: During a standard radical cystectomy in the male, the fine nerves which run along the base of the prostate to the penis are severed, resulting in loss of erections (impotence). If the individual having surgery still has good erections and is sexually active, these nerves can be attempted to be saved by modifying the surgery. Saving the nerves is more difficult to do, it takes more time, and is not always successful.

Female sexual dysfunction: In the female patient at the minimum, the section of the vagina contiguous to the bladder is removed. In the presence of extensive bladder cancer, more of the vagina may need to be removed. Narrowing and shortening of the vagina may result, making sexual intercourse difficult, painful, or impossible. The vagina is reconstructed intraoperatively so that sexual relations can continue. For those requiring major removal of the vagina, future reconstruction of the vagina by additional surgery can be accomplished once the individual has fully recovered and is free of cancer.

Hernia: After surgery, there is an increased risk of developing an incisional hernia (a hernia through the original incision) or an inguinal hernia (a hernia in the groin). A hernia represents a weakening of the thick outer layer of tissue which holds the abdominal contents in place. With a hernia, there is an abnormal protrusion of peritoneal sac and possibly bowel. Herniation of bowel may lead to a lack of blood flow to the herniated intestine which can be serious if left untreated. Surgical correction of the hernia is usually recommended to avoid this possibility and to eliminate discomfort.

Prolonged ileus: For some individuals return of bowel function may be delayed by several days or longer. Your urologist will be following you carefully to make sure a bowel obstruction or bowel leak is not present. Ileus may require leaving the nasogastric tube in to suction off excessive fluid. In addition, hyperalimentation (complete nutrition delivered intravenously) may be initiated if the ileus is prolonged.

Urine leak: The ureters are sewn to the ileal loop in a watertight fashion. In addition, small tubes, called stents, are placed through the ileal loop, through the anastomosis of the ureter to the loop, up the ureter into each kidney. These tubes are placed to allow the ureteral-ileal anastomosis to heal and to prevent leakage. They are generally removed weeks after surgery. Besides these stents, a drain or drains are placed to siphon off any urine which may still leak from the anastomosis. Prolonged urine leakage into the abdomen will generally result in ileus and possibly secondary infection. Persistent urine leak may result from the lack of good blood supply to the ends of the ureters. Leakage is also increased in those who have had pelvic radiation in the past for other malignancies. Prolonged leakage may require repeat surgery.

Wound infection: The rate of wound infection is low. Rates are increased in diabetics, obese individuals, prolonged surgery, and in those individuals whose body temperature drops excessively during surgery. Excellent surgical technique and the use of antibiotics can lower the rate. Wound infections generally will require opening the area to allow drainage. Wound infection can result in weakening of the abdominal closure, which can cause a hernia or more rarely an evisceration (a disruption of the abdominal closure), requiring immediate surgical closure.

Complications common to all surgeries:

Cardiovascular complications: Major surgery can result in significant physical stress to the body and its physiology. Cardiac arrhythmias (abnormal heart beats) may occur and warrant medical therapy to correct. If serious, a cardiologist may be consulted. Life threatening arrhythmias may require cardioversion to correct or even the possibility of a pacemaker. A heart attack (a vascular blockage to the heart) or a cerebrovascular accident also referred to as a stroke, are fortunately rare, but sometimes devastating complications which can prove to be fatal. It is essential an individual facing major surgery with cardiac or vascular disease be properly screened prior to surgery to rule out and correct any serious underlying abnormalities. One should not face surgery with an unstable major underlying condition without correction or improvement when this can be reasonably achieved.

Pulmonary problems: After surgery, it is essential to do deep breathing exercises usually with a device called a spirometer. Bed rest, pain from surgery, and the sedative effects of pain medication can all lead to inadequate aeration of the lungs, which can lead to atelectasis (a collapsed area of the lung). Left untreated, atelectasis can lead to infection (pneumonitis or pneumonia), a potentially serious complication. For those with preceding lung disease, a respiratory therapist will likely be requested to work with the patient to clear lung secretions and increase aeration to prevent infection.

Another potential serious pulmonary problem is called pulmonary embolus. A pulmonary embolus causes damage to the lung by a blood clot which forms in another area of the body, travels through the veins of the body and ends in the lungs. Blood clots can form in the pelvic veins as a result of surgery. They can also form in the lower extremities because of prolonged bed rest and immobility after surgery. Compression stockings used during and after surgery until mobility resumes help to prevent clots in the legs. Getting the individual out of bed and ambulating as soon as possible after surgery are important to prevent clots from forming. In addition, subcutaneous heparin (a medication that stops clotting) can be given during the post-operative period to lessen the possibility of pulmonary embolus without a substantial increase in post-operative bleeding. The symptoms of a pulmonary embolus are shortness of breath and pain in the chest with breathing. Clinical signs include a rapid heart beat and poor oxygenation of the blood. Diagnosis is confirmed with a ventilation-perfusion scan. This study will demonstrate a lack of blood flow in various parts of the lung which have good air flow (a finding consistent with a vascular blockage by a clot). In many institutions, a CT angiogram of the lungs has become the preferred study because of the speed of the study and its enhanced accuracy. An individual must not be allergic to IV contrast, nor have significant renal insufficiency if this test is to be ordered. Pulmonary emboli are usually treated with supportive measures such as supplemental oxygen and anti-coagulation of the blood to prevent further clots from forming and migrating. If a large clot has formed and continues to embolize to the lung, a small filter device may be placed in the main vein of the abdomen (the inferior vena cava) to prevent further clots from traveling to the lungs.

DESPITE DEVELOPING SERIOUS, INVASIVE BLADDER CANCER, I WOULD LIKE TO KEEP MY BLADDER. ARE THERE ANY OTHER OPTIONS OTHER THAN RADICAL CYSTECTOMY?

Complete resection of a small muscle invasive bladder cancer at times can eradicate the cancer. However, diligent follow up with repeat biopsies and repeat resections will be necessary as recurrent disease and further progression are likely. Combination therapy with tumor resection, chemotherapy, and radiation is an additional option, which has proven to be effective in some individuals.

CAN YOU TELL ME MORE ABOUT COMBINATION THERAPY TO SAVE MY BLADDER?

Recently, a number of clinical studies have demonstrated that in select individuals with muscle invasive bladder cancer, utilization of three modes of therapy can be effective in controlling invasive bladder cancer. [1] These bladder preservation protocols have found those individuals that do best have smaller, invasive bladder cancers that can be completely resected. Resection is followed by radiation, which is then followed by chemotherapy. Those that fail the initial treatment go on to cystectomy. Long term bladder preservation in some studies is achieved in approximately 40%. It should be noted however, this high rate of success may be contingent on choosing patients with less serious disease than the average patient undergoing cystectomy. Platinum based chemotherapy appears to offer the best results; however, the best combination regimen of chemotherapy is still being studied. Individuals with large, invasive cancers and those with associated CIS or hydronephrosis secondary to cancer are not considered good candidates for bladder preserving therapy. Side effects of therapy are predominately the effects of chemotherapy, and include nausea, vomiting, diarrhea, fatigue, and sepsis secondary to lowered immunity.

---

[1] Schoenberg M.Management of Invasive and Metastatic Bladder Cancer. Campbell's Urology,Volume 4, 2002; 2810.

CHAPTER ELEVEN
BLADDER SUBSTITUTION

Once the bladder has been removed surgically, the urinary tract must be reconstructed to allow passage of urine from the kidneys to outside the body. This chapter will explore the basics of bladder substitution.

WHAT IS AN ILEAL LOOP, AND WHY IS IT THE MOST COMMON FORM OF URINARY TRACT RECONSTRUCTION?

After removal of the bladder, an approximately 6 inch piece of small intestine from the ileum (the final section of small intestine) is surgically separated from the rest of the small intestine. This section of bowel is used to create an ileal loop diversion. The ileum is the best section of small bowel to use since it has the lowest rate of electrolyte (body salts) disturbances afterwards. The ileum from which this section is removed is reconnected via suturing or staples.

The future ileal loop is flushed clean and the base of the loop is sewn shut. The ends of both ureters are then carefully sewn to a small opening made close to the base of the ileal loop. The opposite end of the ileal loop is brought out through the skin and secured. The end of the loop is everted and tied down to the skin to create a raised stoma. Usually, small plastic tubes called stents are placed through the ileal loop, up the ureters, with their ends curling in the kidneys. These stents are temporary, generally left in for several weeks. Stents serve the purpose of decreasing urinary leakage at the anastomosis (the connection of the ureter to the ileal loop) and serve to allow the anastomosis to heal in an open fashion, thereby reducing the incidence of scarring. The ileal loop is the simplest and quickest form of urinary diversion. Post-operative complications are infrequent. Given these advantages, it remains the most common form of urinary diversion.

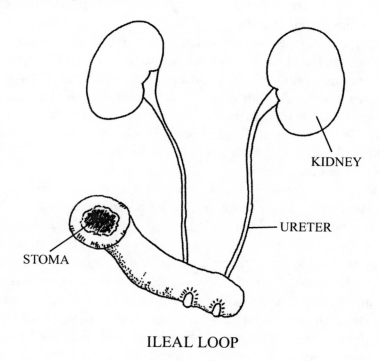

ILEAL LOOP

WHAT IS THE PURPOSE OF THE ILEAL LOOP?

Although one can bring a ureter directly to the skin surface, it is generally not a good form of diversion. The ureters are flimsy, making them prone to obstruction if they are brought out directly. It may also be difficult to bring both ureters to the same place, thus necessitating two drainage bags. The ileal loop serves as a conduit and not a reservoir. The ureters are attached to it at its base. The ileal loop then traverses the skin and underlying tissues to allow unimpeded flow of urine. Urine flows continually through the loop and is collected in a bag attached over the exit of the loop, called the stoma.

WHAT ARE THE COMPLICATIONS THAT CAN OCCUR WHEN ONE HAS AN ILEAL LOOP DIVERSION?

Fortunately, complications are infrequent. The following are the most common complications:

Hernia: During the formation of an ileal loop or continent diversion, the ileal loop is brought out through a peritoneal opening, then through fascia (a thick supporting layer) out through the skin. If a gap exists or develops through the fascia, a parastomal hernia can develop. A hernia represents an abnormal pocket of peritoneum and possibly includes bowel. In addition, a hernia may develop through the surgical incision, which is called an incisional hernia. There is also a higher incidence of inguinal hernia (groin hernia) developing after surgery. Malnutrition, obesity, and lung diseases resulting in labored breathing all increase the risk for a hernia occurring. Many hernias require surgical correction.

Kidney deterioration: If an individual faces recurrent urinary infections involving the kidneys, or has kidney stones, the kidneys may gradually lose function. Fortunately, this complication is rare. Your urologist will aggressively treat urinary infections, stones or deal with other complications which can impair kidney function.

Kidney stones: There is a small but real increased rate of kidney stones after an ileal loop diversion. Kidney stones are most often treated with ESWL (extracoporeal shock wave lithotripsy, a machine that can focus shock waves through the body to break up the stones).

Skin irritation: The skin surrounding the stoma and sometimes the skin beneath the collection bag may become reddened and irritated. By working with your enterostomy nurse, you will learn how to make your ostomy appliance more adherent. Sometimes, application of an ointment to the skin to protect it from the irritating effect of urine is required.

Stomal stenosis: Sometimes the stoma may be too tight, causing urine to pool in the ileal loop, leading to a urinary infection. This can be determined via a loopogram (an X ray study of the loop filled with contrast). Surgical correction of the loop is often required to resolve this problem.

Urinary infection: The ileal loop often can become colonized with bacteria. Colonization does not result in inflammation or any symptoms. However, bacteria may invade the wall of the ileal loop or travel up to the kidneys, resulting in infection. Symptoms may occur, including pain in the loop, kidney pain, blood in the urine, or increased sediment. A fever may occur, especially with kidney infection. To test for infection, urine is collected for culture directly from the loop. Appropriate antibiotics are then used to resolve the infection.

Ureteral-Ileal anastomotic stenosis: The ureters are carefully attached to the base of the ileal loop. Stents are placed at the time of surgery to allow the connection to heal in an open fashion. Nevertheless, the ureteral anastomosis may scar over time, leading to blockage of the ureter and its respective kidney. The kidney becomes swollen with a dilation of its drainage system (hydronephrosis). It is routine to periodically check the condition of the kidneys after ileal loop diversion to make sure the kidneys are not becoming obstructed. Obstruction, if present, will become apparent on follow up studies. If hydronephrosis develops, a loopogram is then obtained. In a normal ileal loop, there should be free reflux of urine up the ureters. If this reflux is gone and the kidney has recently become hydronephrotic, often an anastomotic obstruction has developed. These obstructions can form because of lack of blood flow to the end of the ureter. If the individual has had prior radiation to the pelvis, the rate of blockage is increased. On occasion, obstruction may be secondary to recurrent transitional cell cancer at the end of the ureter. This complication is either handled via an endoscopic method (using a balloon to dilate the ureter or a scope passed to the site and an incision made) or by open surgical revision and correction.

WHAT'S IT LIKE LIVING WITH AN ILEAL LOOP?

After bladder removal surgery, you will first become accustomed to your stoma, and the mechanics of keeping your collection appliance in place. The stoma is composed of the end of ileal loop (urostomy) which is brought out through the skin and everted (folded back) and secured to the skin. The location of the future stoma is usually determined prior to surgery. Ideally, it will be below your "belt line," and definitely away from any skin indentations which can occur from body fat or scars. The stoma is red in appearance, moist, and has no sensation when you touch it. It measures approximately 1-1 ½ inches across and has been described as looking like a "rosebud." It will be the only visible manifestation of your ileal loop diversion.

Getting used to a urostomy takes time. One must overcome issues with altered body image. Realizing the removal of your bladder was necessary to preserve your life, most individuals readily accept the urostomy and its care as the price for surviving and getting on with living.

The next step is to learn how to care for it and the collection appliance. Many individuals now use a collection bag which fits directly over the urostomy with the base of the bag adherent to the surrounding skin, accomplished with a hypoallergenic adhesive. Care of the urostomy can be as simple as gently washing the skin around the stoma and then applying the adhesive bag. A seal can last around four days. Once the seal is deficient, a new bag is applied. Most collection bags snap on and off the underling adhesive base, which makes changing a bag possible without removing the adhesive seal. Depending on your urostomy and your preferences, your enterostomy nurse will work with you to figure out which device works best for you. Some individuals benefit by having an elastic strap secured to the bag and around their waist. Separate stretch belts are also available to help keep the ostomy bag in place.

During the day time, the urine drains directly into the bag attached over the stoma. Bags can either be transparent or opaque. Depending on how much fluid you are drinking and how physically active you are, the bag may need to be drained approximately every four hours. Emptying the bag is accomplished easily by opening the drainage port and allowing the urine to empty directly into a toilet. If you don't want to bother getting up in the middle of the night to drain the bag, the collection bag can be drained via a tube to a larger capacity bed side bag. This bag can be disconnected in the morning from the collection pouch.

Immediately after formation of an ileal loop, there may be much sediment in the urine. This material is a by product of the ileal loop surface lining. Over time, this sediment decreases and with good hydration, the urine takes on a normal appearance.

A urostomy and its collection bag are not apparent under someone's clothing. Usually there is minimal or no odor. An individual with a urostomy can continue to enjoy all physical activities.

WHAT ALTERNATIVES EXIST TO ILEAL LOOP DIVERSION AFTER BLADDER REMOVAL SURGERY?

Alternatives may be considered if an individual prefers not to live with the drainage bag required with an ileal loop. With a continent diversion, a pouch is formed out of bowel beneath the skin. This pouch is extended through the skin and ends with a stoma. This stoma however, does not leak urine continuously into a bag. It requires the individual to catheterize the pouch to drain it.

The other option is called a neobladder. In this technique, a pouch is again formed out of bowel, which is then connected to the individual's urethra. There is no stoma. Catheterization may be required to drain the pouch.

CAN YOU GIVE ME MORE INFORMATION REGARDING A CONTINENT DIVERSION?

In a continent diversion, the urologist creates a pouch out of small bowel, large bowel, or a combination of the two. Through various techniques, a sphincter mechanism is created which makes the pouch continent so that no urine leaks through the stoma. No collection bag therefore is required. Ideally, the pouch eventually can hold 10-15 ounces of urine. Catheterization is required approximately every 4 hours to drain the pouch. There are many surgical techniques to create a continent diversion.

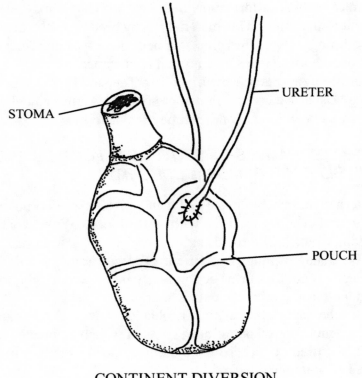

STOMA

URETER

POUCH

CONTINENT DIVERSION

IS EVERYONE WHO HAS THEIR BLADDER REMOVED A CANDIDATE FOR A CONTINENT DIVERSION?

Since urine sits in the pouch until drained by a catheter, there is a higher likelihood of metabolic abnormalities (salt imbalances) occurring compared to the ileal loop, which acts only as a conduit. Therefore, individuals with liver disease or significant renal disease are not candidates. Also, since catheterization is required periodically throughout the day by the individual, the person choosing a continent diversion must have the coordination and motivation to accomplish this.

WHAT ARE THE ADVANTAGES TO HAVING A CONTINENT DIVERSION COMPARED TO AN ILEAL LOOP?

Very simply, one can part with the collection bag. The stoma is cleaned and then catheterized with reusable catheters. Afterwards, the stoma is covered with a dry bandage. For some individuals this is a great advantage. For others, the need to catheterize is not ideal, and they prefer the simplicity of a drainage bag.

WHAT ARE THE DISADVANTAGES RELATED TO A CONTINENT DIVERSION?

The actual surgery to form the continent diversion may take several hours more to accomplish compared to an ileal loop. This additional surgical time is not a problem as long as the individual is in good health, and the surgery has gone well. Not all urologists do continent diversions on a regular basis. If a urologist does not do this operation regularly, you will be better off finding a urologist that does, since complications related to this part of the surgery will be increased by inexperience. Because different techniques exist and the level of expertise and experience of each urologist is different, it is important to ask the urologist about the complications that may occur and the general frequency of occurrence he has seen in his patients. Complications unique to this diversion as compared to the ileal loop may occur, requiring reoperation in up to 20% of patients. If the complication rate is unacceptable, consider an ileal loop. The most common complications are:

Difficulty with catheterization: After the surgery the pouch may become increasingly difficult to empty. Surgical reconstruction is mandatory if a pouch cannot be readily emptied.

Incontinence: During surgery, the continence mechanism is checked. However, at some time after surgery, incontinence may occur, necessitating the wearing of a collection device. In addition, the pouch may still need to be catheterized. Surgical reconstruction is required to reformat the continence mechanism.

Pouch stones: Stones may form in the pouch. Removal may be accomplished with a scope either through the stoma or directly through the skin above the pouch.

PLEASE TELL ME ABOUT THE CREATION OF A NEOBLADDER.

Neobladder means new bladder. In this surgery, the urologist uses a combination of small bowel, large bowel, or a combination of both to create a new bladder pouch which is attached to the remaining urethra. The individual can void by increasing abdominal pressure which is accomplished by holding one's breath and bearing down. There are many surgical techniques to accomplish the formation of a neobladder.

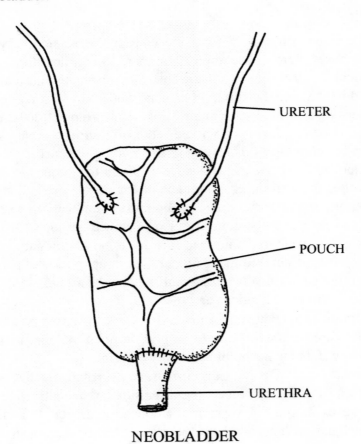

NEOBLADDER

ARE ALL INDIVIDUALS WHO HAVE THEIR BLADDER REMOVED CANDIDATES FOR A NEOBLADDER?

Since urine is stored in a bowel pouch, there is an increased likelihood of metabolic abnormalities occurring compared to the ileal loop, which functions as a conduit. Therefore, those individuals with liver disease or significant renal disease are not candidates. Also, since self catheterization may be required, the individual must have the coordination to accomplish this. Catheterization may be uncomfortable as the catheter is passing through the urethra. The absolute contraindication to the formation of a neobladder is the presence of cancer at the urethral margin. During the cystectomy, the urethral margin is checked by the pathologist for evidence of cancer. If cancer is found at the surgical margin, a urethrectomy is performed, and a continent diversion or ileal loop is accomplished for diversion.

WHAT ARE THE DISADVANTAGES OF HAVING A NEOBLADDER?

There are a number of issues which need to be reviewed. Cancer recurrence in the urethra after the formation of a neobladder would likely require surgery to remove the urethra and a new form of urinary diversion. After cystectomy, urethral recurrence of cancer can be expected in approximately 10% of patients. Those with multi-focal disease and especially with disease near the bladder neck will likely have a higher recurrence rate in the urethra. For those with a neobladder, the urethra must be carefully followed for possible cancer recurrence. Monitoring is accomplished by washings of the urethra for cytology or by visual inspection with a scope. If there is a concern for an increased risk of urethral recurrence given the nature of the individual's bladder cancer, the formation of a neobladder should be avoided.

Urinary incontinence may occur after the formation of the neobladder because of damage to the continence mechanism of the urethra. The nerves to the urethral sphincter travel deep in the pelvis and generally are not injured during surgery. However, meticulous care must be taken in handling the urethra and the sphincter muscle around it. Complications resulting in scar tissue may also jeopardize the continence mechanism leading to leakage. Marked scarring between the neobladder and the urethra may occur, but is readily handled via an incision or dilation of the blockage accomplished through a cystoscope. Even in those with an intact sphincter, especially in females, leakage often occurs at night, necessitating the wearing of a pad.

For some individuals, the neobladder is not adequately emptied with increased abdominal pressure. The solution is intermittent self catheterization through the native urethra. This can be uncomfortable, especially for male patients. For many individuals continence is preserved and catheterization is not required, making this an excellent form of diversion.

Creating a neobladder is technically more difficult and will require several more hours of surgery as compared to the simpler ileal loop diversion. Many urologists do not create neobladders on a regular basis. If your urologist does not do this part of the operation frequently, you are better off finding a urologist who does neobladder surgery regularly or you will face the prospect of a higher complication rate. It is important to question your urologist regarding the various complications and the frequency of occurrence he has seen in his patients. Ideally, the individual with a neobladder will empty without the need for catheterization and will remain continent between emptying. It is important to understand what percentage of individuals can expect this ideal outcome. If the probability for incontinence or need to catheterize is too high a risk for you, choose a continent diversion or an ileal loop diversion instead.

CHAPTER TWELVE
TREATMENT OF METASTATIC
BLADDER CANCER

In this chapter, we review the basics of therapy for bladder cancer which has spread or is likely to spread beyond the confines of the bladder and possibly throughout the body (metastatic cancer).

MY UROLOGIST HAS REFERRED ME TO AN ONCOLOGIST FOR TREATMENT. WHY DOESN'T MY UROLOGIST GIVE ME CHEMOTHERAPY?

Your urologist is a surgical specialist in diseases of the genitourinary system. A physician who specializes in treating cancer with chemotherapy is called an oncologist. These physicians are cancer specialists who are expert in choosing, delivering, and monitoring patients who are given chemotherapy to assure the best possible outcome. Your oncologist will play a crucial role in guiding you through the intricacies of chemotherapy. It is essential to have a specialist skilled in using chemotherapy to treat you.

HOW IMPORTANT IS IT TO HAVE AN EXCELLENT ONCOLOGIST?

It is critical to have a top notch oncologist, knowledgeable in the most effective chemotherapy regimens, and diligent in his care of you. Chemotherapy agents have potentially serious side effects, some life threatening. Your oncologist is responsible for getting you through these regimens with the least possible side effects and risks. In addition, these therapies can be particularly taxing. It is essential that your oncologist be a compassionate physician who can team with you during this phase of your therapy. He must be willing to take the time to discuss the proposed therapy, its risks and alternatives. A complete discussion regarding potential success of therapy, versus side effects and risks should be a key part of any consultation for chemotherapy.

WHAT EXACTLY IS CHEMOTHERAPY AND HOW DOES IT WORK?

Chemotherapy uses drugs to kill cancer. There are many different types of chemotherapy. Some drugs work better than others for specific cancers. Some are given orally as pills. Many are given intravenously. Susceptibility to chemotherapy varies depending on the specific cancer. Some, like testicular cancer, are extremely sensitive to chemotherapy while others, like kidney cancer, are not. Bladder cancer is felt to be moderately sensitive to chemotherapy.

Chemotherapy drugs work systemically, throughout the body. These drugs work via various mechanisms to damage and hopefully kill rapidly dividing cells. Since cancer cells are for the most part rapidly dividing, they are generally sensitive to chemotherapy. Other rapidly dividing cells in the body may also suffer injury during chemotherapy, which is why people often experience hair loss, anemia, and diarrhea as a result of therapy. Chemotherapy also can lower the blood cells that fight infection, leading to a diminished immune system and an increased susceptibility for acquiring a potentially serious infection.

WHEN IS CHEMOTHERAPY USED IN BLADDER CANCER?

Chemotherapy is offered most often in the face of metastatic disease or advanced local disease that cannot be removed surgically. Chemotherapy in this setting can result in complete response (disappearance of all visible tumors) in approximately 20% of patients. For these individuals, success of therapy can be monitored with imaging studies such as CT scans. Despite initial improvement, long term survival is rare.

Neoadjuvant therapy, therapy given prior to cystectomy, has several advantages. Chemotherapy is given to the patient prior to surgery when the person is strongest. Tumors can be reduced in size potentially making surgery easier when dealing with larger cancers. Earlier treatment of micro-metastatic disease may offer improved results. Most studies have demonstrated the regimens to be well tolerated and do not increase surgical complications afterwards. The downside is the delay of surgery by approximately three months which can be critical for patients whose chemotherapy is ineffective. In addition, one must face the toxicities of this therapy which may affect the individual's overall state of health prior to surgery. Since the true pathologic stage is unknown, many patients with organ confined disease may receive chemotherapy unnecessarily. Many oncologists reserve neoadjuvant therapy for those with disease beyond the bladder (Stage T3 or T4). Some studies have shown a reduction in mortality, while others have not. One recent article which reviewed multiple studies using neoadjuvant cisplatin based combination therapy showed a 6.5% improved survival at 5 years.[1]

Adjuvant therapy is chemotherapy given after cystectomy and complete removal of all visible cancer. This form of therapy is generally reserved for those with disease outside the bladder (Stage T3 or T4). Since the actual pathologic stage is available, unnecessary chemotherapy for those with organ confined cancer is avoided. However, there is no visible tumor to be followed on imaging studies making it impossible to determine whether or not initial progress is being made. Given the limited number of studies available, there may be some benefit of adjuvant therapy in a select group of patients at high risk of recurrence. Although time to progression is prolonged,

[1]   Advanced Bladder Cancer Meta-analysis Collaboration: Neoadjuvant chemotherapy in invasive bladder cancer: a systematic review and meta-analysis. Lancet 361: 1927, 2003.

it is not clear if long term survival is improved.[2] Since there are no great survival differences to receiving neoadjuvant versus adjuvant therapy, some may argue that if adjuvant therapy is to be given, it makes sense to deliver it after surgery. This has the added advantage of having available post-operatively a complete pathologic staging, allowing for more proper selection of those most likely to benefit from chemotherapy.

WHAT CHEMOTHERAPY IS GIVEN FOR METASTATIC BLADDER CANCER?

The most common regimen consists of using four different drugs MVAC (methotrexate, vinblastine, adriamycin and cisplatin) given in a 21 or 28 day cycle. During each cycle, different chemotherapy drugs are given on different days to afford maximal cancer killing effect and minimizing side effects. Generally, two cycles are given prior to assessing effectiveness and proceeding with further chemotherapy.

WHAT ARE THE MOST EFFECTIVE DRUGS FOR BLADDER CANCER?

Historically, the most effective drug regimen and the standard of care is MVAC. This combination of drugs is more effective than any drug alone. The drug regimen consists of methotrexate, vinblastine, adriamycin, and cisplatin. This regimen is difficult to tolerate. Side effects and toxicities include nausea, diarrhea, bone marrow suppression (resulting in anemia and a drop in the white blood cells, which fight infection, a drop in platelets, which help in clotting, mouth ulcers, the possibility of kidney and heart damage, and nerve impairment resulting in numbness). Because of the decline in the immune system as a result of this regimen, serious infection leading to death occurs in approximately 3% of patients. Given the serious side effects and potential for the possibility of life threatening complications, only an experienced oncologist should supervise this

---

[2]   Stockle, M., Wellek, S., Meyenburg,W., Voges, G.E., Fischer, U.,Gertenbach, U. et al: Radical cystectomy with or without adjuvant polychemotherapy for non-organ-confined transitional cell carcinoma of the urinary bladder: prognostic impact of lymph node involvement. Urology, 48:868, 1996.

therapy. By careful monitoring and the use of medications to control side effects, the therapy can be made safer and easier to tolerate.

For the elderly or those individuals not in the best of health, gemcitabine combined with cisplatin (GC) have become an effective, but less toxic combination. This therapy was not originally believed to be as effective as MVAC, but is more tolerable and does not have the higher risk of serious secondary infections developing. A recent randomized trial compared MVAC with GC. In this study of 405 patients, an overall response of approximately 50% was seen with either regimen, with substantially lower toxicity with GC.[3] Although the study cannot predict overall differences in survival, the similar response rate with reduction in toxicity has now made GC first line therapy for an increasing number of oncologists.

HOW EFFECTIVE IS CHEMOTHERAPY IN METASTATIC BLADDER CANCER?

Initial response as noted above occurs in approximately 50% of individuals with metastatic bladder cancer treated with first line combination chemotherapy. Those with more advanced disease generally have a more limited response and more rapid progression. Unfortunately, long term disease free survival is rare.

Some individuals may have cancer which is initially too advanced to surgically remove. After treatment with chemotherapy, reduction of tumor may occur, allowing surgical removal of the remaining cancer with the potential for disease free survival. [4]

---

[3] von der Maase, H., Hansen, S.W., Roberts, J.T., Dogliotti, L., Oliver, T., Moore, M. J. et al: Gemcitabine and Cisplatin versus methotrexate, vinblastine, doxorubicin and cisplatin in advanced or metastatic bladder cancer: results of a large, randomized, multinational, multicenter, phase III study. J Clin Oncol, 17: 3068, 2000.

[4] Herr, H. W., Donat, S. M. and Bajorin, D.F.: Post-chemotherapy surgery in patients with unresectable or regionally metastatic bladder cancer. J Urol,165, 811, 2001.

HOW IS CHEMOTHERAPY GIVEN?

Chemotherapy is given via an intravenous line usually placed at the time of medication administration. For those individuals that lack usable peripheral veins, an intravenous line can be placed into a larger, more central vein. These lines require more effort to place, but can be kept in place for weeks and utilized for many courses of chemotherapy. The chemotherapy medication is infused directly into the vein with minimal or no discomfort.

WILL I NEED SOMEONE TO DRIVE ME TO AND FROM APPOINTMENTS FOR CHEMOTHERAPY?

Since most individuals will experience nausea and often weakness from chemotherapy, it is wise to have someone drive you to and from your appointment. If after several treatments you find you tolerate the therapy without any marked initial side effects, you may choose to drive yourself.

WHAT PRECAUTIONS WILL I NEED TO TAKE AFTER CHEMOTHERAPY?

After chemotherapy, you will generally be extremely tired and weak. Getting the rest you need, eating a healthy diet once nausea subsides, and staying well hydrated are key to your recovery from the side effects of chemotherapy. Your oncologist will provide you with medication to combat side effects. You should also have an understanding of which side effects are potentially serious and when you are to call your oncologist.

Since your blood counts will be lowered temporarily, it is important to stay away from individuals who have viral or bacterial infections that are contagious. It is essential you deal with any persistent emotional stress or depression which may occur from your illness and treatment as these can lower your immune system. A healthy immune system is necessary for good health. Talk to your oncologist, urologist, or primary care physician if you need help. Confide with your spouse, loved one, friend, or clergy for support. Participating in a cancer support group may be beneficial. Don't isolate yourself from others as their support may be critical for your recovery.

ARE THERE SOME PATIENTS WITH METASTATIC BLADDER CANCER WHO ARE NOT CANDIDATES FOR CHEMOTHERAPY?

The elderly, frail individuals with multiple coexisting chronic illnesses, individuals that are weakened through malnutrition or who have compromised immunity all would face substantially increased risk of complications from standard chemotherapy regimens for bladder cancer. Unfortunately, cisplatin is toxic to kidneys, and many individuals with bladder cancer have compromised kidney function which effectively rules out the use of platinum based chemotherapy. Other treatment regimens exist and are being worked on for these individuals, but none show the efficacy of the standard therapy which includes cisplatin.

ARE THERE ANY OTHER TREATMENT REGIMENS AVAILABLE IF INITIAL CHEMOTHERAPY FAILS?

Most individuals treated with standard chemotherapy regimens with metastatic bladder cancer will have recurrence and progression of their disease. Multiple treatment regimens have been utilized with overall response rates of 10-40%.[5] To date, regimens have generally used taxanes, both docetaxel and paclitaxel. Ifosfamide has been shown to have significant single agent activity as well, but is extremely toxic. Combination therapy with taxanes and ifosfamide are presently being tested.

MY FAMILY HAS ENCOURAGED ME TO GO TO A CANCER CENTER FOR EXPERIMENTAL THERAPY, SHOULD I?

This can only be answered based on your individual history of cancer care, your health status, and the present state of your cancer. Experimental therapy is just that; it is still in the investigational stage

[5] Rosenberg, JE, Carroll, Peter R., Small, Eric J, Update on Chemotherapy for Advanced Bladder Cancer. J Urol, 174: 18, 2005.

and has not yet been determined whether or not it is completely safe and or effective. A patient may or may not qualify to be in a cancer trial depending on age and other risk factors, stage of cancer, or prior therapy.

During phase 1 of a cancer trial, the safety of the chemotherapy dose is being determined. During the early part of the trial, a lower dose may be used. The dose is gradually increased to determine the potential for side effects. Individuals entering the trial later may receive higher doses, more potentially serious side effects, and not necessarily more effective therapy. During phase 2, it is determined how often a particular cancer will respond to the chemotherapy at a fixed dose regimen. Lastly, during phase 3, the new drug which appears to be effective is compared to the current accepted chemotherapy for a particular cancer.

This brief review undermines the uncertainty of receiving chemotherapy during an experimental protocol. If the individual needs chemotherapy, it is generally safer and wiser to receive the standard regimen already established as safe and possibly effective. If however, prior standard chemotherapy has proven to be ineffective, or if the patient cannot tolerate standard therapy and the patient's health allows for additional chemo, enrollment in a chemotherapy trial may be appropriate if the individual qualifies. At times, there can be breakthroughs and new agents can be more effective in eradicating cancer than the established drugs.

I AM CONCERNED BY THE TOXICITIES OF CHEMOTHERAPY. SHOULD I GO THROUGH WITH IT?

The answer to this question must always be an individual one. It is best answered after considering the potential gain versus the potential side effects and risks.

Initial side effects experienced by almost all individuals will include nausea and vomiting, diarrhea, mouth ulcers, extreme fatigue, loss of appetite and weight loss, hair loss, and a drop in blood counts. Many of the side effects can be lessened by taking appropriate medication. Long term side effects include low blood count, nerve and kidney damage. Side effects can be severe and potentially life threatening. Death as the result of sepsis from MVAC treatment occurs in approximately 3% of patients. Even if side effects are not severe, chemotherapy may result in the individual rapidly becoming weak and tired, reducing markedly his quality of life. The side effects for the most part are not long lasting with a return to normalcy after chemotherapy has been completed. If you are not tolerating the chemotherapy regimen well, your oncologist can modify the dose, frequency of dosing, or alter the regimen entirely.

When facing the prospects of chemotherapy, it is essential to have an oncologist who can inform you fully of the potential probable effectiveness of the chemotherapy being offered. Just as importantly, the toxicities of the chemotherapy must be fully reviewed. Of course, there are no absolutes when reviewing the potential for success and failure. Each individual's cancer is unique. Some respond better than others to chemotherapy. General statistics regarding disease regression and remission are available. Absolute numbers for the individual are not.

After several courses of chemotherapy, an assessment of your clinical progress will be made. This will generally require a study such as a CAT scan, to check the response of the cancer to the chemotherapy. If progress is being made and the individual is tolerating the chemotherapy, a decision is then made to continue the chemotherapy to completion. If on the other hand, the cancer is not responding or the individual is not tolerating the therapy, a decision can be made to stop further chemotherapy, alter the present regimen, or try a different course of chemotherapy.

As new drugs are introduced and new combinations of drugs are tested, statistics regarding effectiveness are constantly changing. Side effects too can vary, depending on the individual. However, most patients will experience the side effects to various degrees, and these need to be fully understood prior to proceeding.

In the end, it is the individual's decision as to whether to begin or end chemotherapy. For many, trying chemo and seeing the effect on the cancer is a sound decision. If the cancer does not respond or if the patient finds the side effects unacceptable, chemotherapy can be stopped. It is extremely important for you to have an oncologist who will work with you closely. Your oncologist should understand your feelings regarding cancer treatment fully. The importance of fighting for prolongation of life versus the treatments' effect on your quality of life should be part of your initial and ongoing discussions with your oncologist.   Sharing your concerns with your oncologist will go a long way in allaying your fears and allowing you to make the best possible decision for yourself.

CHAPTER THIRTEEN
TREATMENT FOR ERECTILE DYSFUNCTION

In this chapter we will explore erectile dysfunction, a common problem for men with bladder cancer.

WHAT IS ERECTILE DYSFUNCTION?

This condition was previously referred to as impotence. Erectile dysfunction better describes a condition which has many causes and has varied manifestations. In brief, erectile dysfunction refers to the inability of a man to obtain and maintain an erection sufficient to have sexual intercourse on a regular basis. Although sexual dysfunction involves much more than the quality of the man's erection, this chapter will focus on this aspect since it is so often a side effect of major cancer surgery.

WHAT ARE THE MECHANICS OF AN ERECTION?

When the genitals are stimulated directly or the male has either a visual or mental erotic experience, nerve impulses are increased to the penis, resulting in the relaxation of muscle fibers within the vascular chambers of the penis called the corpora cavernosa. These chambers then become engorged with blood, resulting in a firm or erect penis. During the filling of the corpora cavernosa, the drainage veins of the penis are occluded. Testosterone, known as the male hormone, is necessary for sexual desire (libido) and for the proper sexual function of the penis. To obtain a good erection, the individual must have adequate nerve function, sufficient arterial flow into the penis, corpora cavernosa which are pliable, and veins which can be occluded during the filling phase. In addition, the male must not have "performance anxiety" which can prevent the formation and maintenance of an erection.

HOW DOES RADICAL CYSTECTOMY CAUSE ERECTILE DYSFUNCTION?

During the removal of the bladder and prostate, the fine nerves which travel alongside the prostate to the penis are readily damaged. If the nerves are completely severed, permanent erectile dysfunction is the result. If there is partial damage, recovery may occur.

CAN NERVE DAMAGE BE PREVENTED DURING RADICAL CYSTECTOMY?

The neurovascular bundles which run adjacent and adherent to the prostate can be pushed aside as the bladder and prostate are removed. This is more technically difficult compared to the standard non-nerve sparing approach. Sparing the nerves is not always possible even with the best effort. If the individual has questionable erections prior to the surgery, a nerve sparing procedure rarely leads to preservation of erections and therefore is not warranted. Extensive bladder cancer may encroach on the prostate, making a nerve sparing procedure extremely difficult if not impossible.

MY UROLOGIST DID A NERVE SPARING TECHNIQUE. HOW QUICKLY CAN I EXPECT MY ERECTIONS TO RETURN?

There are multiple factors which must be considered. Generally younger patients, those in better overall health, and those with excellent preoperative erections can expect a more rapid return of erectile activity if the nerve sparing approach is successful. Even with meticulous nerve sparing, some nerve injury, either temporary or permanent may occur. The extent of the injury will determine how quickly erections may return. Erections may start returning in as little as two to three months, or may gradually return over a period of a year, or may not return at all.

IS THERE ANY TREATMENT WHICH MAY HELP MY ERECTIONS RETURN SOONER?

It has recently been shown that men who take low dose Viagra on a daily basis after nerve sparing surgery will see there erectile ability return earlier.[1]

HOW DO THE PILLS FOR ERECTILE DYSFUNCTION WORK?

At the present time, three oral medications are available for erectile dysfunction: Viagra, Levitra, and Cialis. All three medications work by increasing and preserving the level of the neurotransmitter active in the penis. It is the neurotransmitter which keeps the nerves active in stimulating the corpora cavernosa to relax and fill with blood. For these medications to work, at least some of the nerves to the penis must be intact. If all the nerves have been damaged beyond recovery, these medications will be ineffective. If erections fail to return over a one year period, it is probable nerve damage is irreparable.

When effective, these medications work quickly, within thirty minutes to an hour. If these medications work, this will be your simplest form of therapy. The medications do not give the individual a spontaneous erection. They simply increase the ability for the patient with dysfunction to obtain an erection. Eventually, erectile activity may return to the point where medication is no longer required.

These medications are contraindicated if you are on nitrates (medications for angina, a condition caused by blockage of the arteries to the heart). The combination of nitrates with these medications can result in a dangerous drop in blood pressure. There are other potential contraindications which will be discussed by your urologist

---

[1] Rupesh Raina, Milton M. Lakin, Ashok Agarwal, Edward Mascha, Drogo K. Montague, Eric Klein, Craig D. Zippe: Efficacy and Factors Associated With Successful Outcome of Sildenafil Citrate Use For Erectile Dysfunction After Radical Prostatectomy; Urology 63 (5) 960-965,2004.

with you. Most common side effects of these medications include flushing, headaches, and temporary alteration of color vision.

WHAT OTHER ALTERNATIVES EXIST FOR TREATMENT OF ERECTILE DYSFUNCTION?

A number of other options are available if oral medications are ineffective, if the individual does not tolerate the medications, or is not a candidate for taking them.

Intracavernosal injections: There are a number of medications which can be injected directly into the corpora to induce an erection. The medications cause relaxation of the muscle in the corpora cavernosa, which allows blood to fill the corpora, resulting in an erection. This technique is accomplished with a small syringe and needle. There is usually minimal discomfort. Most men will get a good erection in a few minutes, ideally lasting approximately one hour. Your urologist will determine the proper dose and teach you how to self inject during a few office visits. Most men can learn the technique readily.

Intraurethral medication: Muse is the product name for a delivery device and medication in pellet form which is squeezed into the urethra. It works by directly relaxing the corporal muscle, which allows blood to fill the corpora, resulting in an erection. It is important to first urinate to lubricate the urethra. The medication is gradually absorbed through the urethra and into the corpora, resulting in an erection. Testing for drug tolerance and dosing are required in the physician's office. Many individuals will experience some burning discomfort in the urethra from the medication. A small percentage of individuals may experience a drop in blood pressure which can lead to passing out. Careful testing of dose and tolerance are therefore required.

Vacuum pump device: A number of vacuum pumps are available without a prescription. Your urologist usually can provide you with information. These devices consist of a plastic cylinder placed over the penis and a battery or hand operated pump to create a vacuum around the penis. The vacuum results in the gradual filling of the corpora cavernosa with blood. Generation of an erection generally takes about 5 minutes. To maintain an erection, a plastic ring is placed around the base of penis for up to 30 minutes. These devices are easy to work and safe to operate. Some patients think they are terrific and others complain about the loss of spontaneity and discomfort from the constricting ring required to maintain an erection.

Penile implant: A number of different implants are available to restore erections. The two main types of devices are the semi-rigid and the inflatable implants. With the semi-rigid device, the erection is induced by the firm, but bendable rods which are placed directly into each corporal body. The individual with such an implant will have a penis which is always semi-erect. The inflatable device allows for a more flaccid appearing penis when not in operation. With this device, fluid is transferred from a reservoir into the penile cylinders to create an erection. After sexual relations, a valve is squeezed to allow the cylinders to drain back into the reservoir resulting in flaccidity. Penile prosthesis can restore full erections. For some individuals, they prove to be the solution if other alternatives are not effective or suitable. There is a small chance the prosthesis can become infected after the surgery, usually requiring removal of the device and eradication of infection prior to reimplantation. With the inflatable device, there is an approximately 5% chance of eventual device failure, making it nonfunctional, requiring repeat surgery for revision.

CHAPTER FOURTEEN
COMPLEMENTARY MEDICINE

This chapter will explore the increased popularity of non-traditional medical therapies. Some reviews have indicated the majority of cancer patients use these therapies at some time during their cancer treatment.

WHAT IS THE DIFFERENCE BETWEEN COMPLEMENTARY AND ALTERNATIVE MEDICINE?

These terms have been often used interchangeably. They utilize non-traditional treatments that have not been incorporated into conventional medical care. These therapies are varied and include herbal medicines, acupuncture, energy healing, and various forms of meditation. It is best not to reject traditional medicine and have it replaced by alternative therapies. Instead, utilizing these non-traditional therapies in conjunction with traditional care makes sense for many. Combining conventional care with complementary care can enhance the patient's well-being and possibly his outcome.

AREN'T HERBAL REMEDIES GENERALLY LESS TOXIC AND POSSIBLY MORE EFFECTIVE THAN TRADITIONAL MEDICINES SINCE THEY COME FROM NATURAL SOURCES?

The popularity of herbal medications has increased dramatically over the past decade. In your local pharmacy one can now find shelves filled with herbal medicines. First, it should be understood approximately 50% of modern medications are derived from plant extracts. Conventional medications are manufactured under strict government scrutiny. Their purity, potency, dosage and safety are all standardized prior to approval. Potential toxicities and drug interactions with other medications are readily available.

Contrast this with herbal remedies. There is at present no government regulation as these remedies are considered supplements. Their purity, potency and strength, and safety are not standardized, nor has their potential toxicities and drug interactions been made readily available. Lately, this has begun to change. Recently the FDA (Food and Drug Administration) took action against a supplement used as a weight loss remedy, but which increased the risk of stroke. The FDA pulled products with this ingredient from circulation. Of course, traditional medications also have substantial risks. The FDA has much better oversight however, with continuous monitoring of drug toxicities in place. On occasion, a conventional medication may be pulled out of circulation, such as the recent realization two drugs used in combination for appetite suppression caused serious heart abnormalities. It must be emphasized that just because a remedy is "natural" or plant based, does not mean it is free of potential toxicity. Since herbal medications can interact with traditional medications, resulting in enhancement or diminishment of the effectiveness of medications, or possibly a toxic interaction, it is important to inform your physicians of any herbal remedies you have been taking. Also, let your urologist know of any herbal medicines you are taking prior to surgery as some may affect blood clotting.

IS THERE ANY ROLE FOR HERBAL REMEDIES IN THE SERIOUSLY ILL CANCER PATIENT?

Some herbs have been shown to be safe and effective to relieve the nausea and the stress associated with cancer treatment. Other herbs claim to improve your immune system or sense of well-being. Many resources are now available to physicians to ascertain the safety and possible use for herbal remedies. As these remedies are used and eventually tested through scientific studies, many may become accepted by physicians and become part of conventional medicine. For the present, make sure you obtain your herbal remedies only from the most reputable sources. Discuss with your physicians what herbs you are taking to make sure they are not reducing the effectiveness of traditional treatment or possibly increasing your risk of a serious side effect or adverse occurrence.

AREN'T SOME OF THESE THERAPIES REALLY JUST A PLACEBO EFFECT?

The placebo effect has been well documented as part of the practice of modern medicine. The placebo effect is pervasive. We humans can feel better or worse depending on our perceptions and expectations, and interactions with others. This effect is so common our current scientific studies are structured so neither the patient nor the clinician knows whether or not the individual receiving the experimental drug or therapy is getting the real treatment or just the placebo (a sugar pill or therapy without merit). The placebo effect is not only a perception within the brain, but results in biochemical changes in the body affecting heart rate, blood pressure, and the function of internal organs.

Many complementary therapies may use the placebo effect to full advantage. So too, the wise physician understands the power of comforting words and a caring demeanor. Providing hope to the individual is powerful medicine. The physician's optimistic attitude and expectation of improvement for the patient is a powerful elixir in itself.

A recent study published in *Science* explored the placebo effect. [1] In this study, individuals received either electric shots or heat applied to their arms. The level of pain was recorded while the subject's brains were monitored via an MRI. Next, the same individuals were told a cream applied to their arms would help block the pain of the same stimuli. The cream was actually ordinary skin cream with no pain relief benefit. Once again, either heat or electric shocks were delivered. MRI was again used. Researchers found that a specific area in the brain was activated by the expectation of pain relief. This resulted in the reduction in brain activity in the area sensing pain and in a reduction in perceived pain. The testing was again repeated, but this time the individuals were told the cream was a placebo. Pain activity in the brain increased and pain perception was back to a high level. This study demonstrates scientifically the power of the placebo effect.

Because they have not been studied scientifically, it is difficult to ascertain whether or not there is more to some complementary therapies than the placebo effect. However, not knowing does not translate to any other effect. We simply do not know. Nevertheless, even if we are dealing with just the placebo effect, this is still a real form of therapy which can improve the quality of a patient's life.

IS ACUPUNCTURE BENEFICIAL?

Acupuncture is an ancient Eastern therapy which involves the insertion of fine acupuncture needles into the body's meridians. These meridians are thought to represent the energy pathways of the body. This practice and the concept behind it are not part of Western medicine. Thus far, randomized control studies have not been able to demonstrate convincing evidence of pain relief beyond the placebo effect. However, a recent controlled study utilized Positron Emission Tomography (PET) to monitor brain activity during sham treatment and real acupuncture treatment. During sham treatment brain activity was increased in an area of the brain which produces natural opiates to reduce pain, confirming the power of the placebo

---

[1]   T.D. Wager et al: Placebo Induced Changes in MRI in the Anticipation and Experience of Pain, Science (303) 1162-1167, 2/20/2004.

effect. With real acupuncture an additional area of the brain involved with pain modulation and thought to be associated with acupuncture treatment was activated, demonstrating a potentially enhanced ability for acupuncture to provide pain relief.[2]

WHAT ABOUT ENERGY HEALING?

Reiki is an ancient Eastern form of healing provided by trained practioners to harmonize the energy flow throughout the body. An individual can learn the technique and practice Reiki on himself regularly to maximize its benefit. This complementary technique can bring a sense of calmness and muscle relaxation to the individual facing a life threatening illness.

I HAVE HEARD OF THE MIND, BODY CONNECTION. IS THIS REAL AND HOW CAN I HARNESS IT TO IMPROVE MY CONDITION?

The mind body connection has recently come under greater scientific scrutiny and curiosity. We are all familiar with the racing heart beat, the sweaty palms, and the tremulous voice characterizing the ever familiar "stage fright." Given a perceived threat, the brain sends out chemical messengers to the body, resulting in very real physical symptoms and signs.

The mind body connection is very real. Chronic stress and anxiety and other negative emotions are thought to potentially damage the immune system. A mental state of calm may enhance it.

Techniques such as guided imagery, meditation, and tai chi are used to calm the brain and potentially enhance the body's ability to fight cancer and heal. How powerful an effect is uncertain given the lack of good studies. At the least, these techniques can improve the patient's quality of life.

---

[2]   Pariente, Jeremie et al: Expectancy and belief modulate the neuronal substrates of pain treated by acupuncture, NeuroImage, Vol 25, Issue 4, 1161-1167, 5/01/2005.

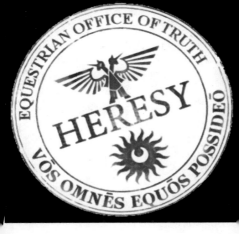

My purity I swear
until the day I die,
My soul I shall not bare
except to Pinkie Pie

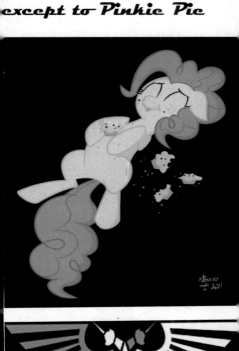

WHAT ABOUT CANCER SUPPORT GROUPS?

Some of the earlier studies showed improved patient outcomes for those that participated in cancer support groups. More recently, studies have not confirmed this. However, for those participating, often there was a real reduction in stress and fear associated with dealing with cancer. These groups serve as a valuable resource for the individual facing so many new unknowns. For some, a formal cancer support group may not be desired. Having a supportive spouse, family member, friend, or clergy can be extremely helpful for the individual dealing with cancer. Sharing your concerns and fears with another can be therapeutic in itself.

HOW ABOUT DIET? IS THERE ANY TRUTH THAT SOME FOODS CAN FIGHT CANCER?

Only recently have foods been intensely studied as potential cancer fighters. For some cancers, a strong link to diet has been found. Prostate, breast, and colon cancer are highly linked to diet. Bladder cancer has a less definite known association. Preliminary studies have shown a possible reduction in recurrence of bladder cancer with a reduction in saturated fats, increased consumption of fruits and vegetables, and taking antioxidant vitamins. The American Cancer Society has a new book entitled, Eating Well, Staying Well During and After Cancer. This book provides information on research related to nutrition and cancer, and provides coping strategies for those challenged with eating and digestion related side effects from cancer. The 288 page paperback book (ISBN 0-944235-51-4) is available through the ACS online at www.cancer.org (click on "Bookstore") or by calling 1-800-ACS-2345.

WHAT ABOUT EXERCISE?

Exercise will improve your heart and lung function, increases your muscle tone, and helps keep your weight down. Exercise can make you feel good too. A number of studies have shown improved brain function and a lessened risk of dementia with regular exercise. These benefits should provide enough justification for all individuals to exercise regularly. How much the immune system is enhanced, and whether or not exercise will improve your cancer prognosis is unfortunately unknown.

In addition to exercise, sleep is important. The body needs sufficient sleep and relaxation to reenergize and face the increased challenges a cancer diagnosis brings.

I'M FEELING REALLY DOWN. I DON'T WANT TO DO ANYTHING. I HAVE LOST MY WILL TO LIVE. IS THIS A COMMON REACTION TO CANCER?

Facing a life threatening cancer can bring on feelings of anxiety and fear. Hopelessness and despair leading to depression is unfortunately a common occurrence. Depression can be devastating. It may sap an individual's energy, which is necessary to live with and survive cancer. If you are not coping well with your cancer and depression persists, it is essential to have a discussion with your physician. For many, medication can rebalance the altered chemistry of the brain, rapidly clearing depression and bringing a new lease on life.

CAN I FIND PEACE AND ENJOY MY LIFE EVEN IF I CAN'T BE CURED OF MY CANCER?

Unfortunately, not all individuals can be cured of their cancer. Many must face this prospect. Some eventually find peace and equanimity, despite facing the inevitable decline which comes from progressive cancer. I have witnessed many individuals with a deep faith that keeps them going through their difficult times. They never seem to lose their sense of peace. For some, it is their faith that an afterlife exists which keeps them at peace. For others, it appears to be a gratitude for a life well lived, without regrets. Some carry old baggage filled with hurts and regrets. They may be angry at friends and relatives for real or misinterpreted grievances. Forgiveness can bring release and bring a new sense of peace. I have talked to patients stricken with terminal cancer who have expressed their appreciation for their illness. They have realized a new, richer understanding of the gift their life has been. Knowing their life is coming to an end, they have let go of old anxieties. They have been able to focus on the love they have for their relatives and friends. They have come to understand the inter relatedness we all have with each other. They have found comfort in finally understanding the meaning of their lives. Although they have not been cured of their cancer, they have found the path to heal themselves.

CHAPTER FIFTEEN
ADVANCE CARE PLANNING

Each of us may eventually face the prospect of an incurable disease. Our mental state may deteriorate to the point where we can no longer have the ability to make health care decisions. It is essential to make your desires known in a legal document to prevent needless medical care which may serve only to prolong the dying process. Facing a hopeless outcome, each of us should have available a living will, a document which details our wishes and desires regarding end of life care. Also, by providing a trusted individual with the power to make medical decisions for you if you become incapacitated, a durable power of attorney, your wishes can be followed involving other aspects of your care. An advance directive includes both these legal documents which detail your preferences for medical care. Facing this difficult topic in the midst of the emotional turmoil of rapidly failing health is extremely difficult. A frank discussion with your loved ones long before you need these documents will assure your wishes are followed and will reduce the possibility of turmoil for your family and health care providers if your wishes are not known.

WHAT IS A LIVING WILL?

This document gives specific instructions to your physician regarding the possibility of withholding life sustaining treatment in the face of a terminal illness or if you are permanently comatose when there is no hope of recovery.

WHAT IS A LIFE SUSTAINING TREATMENT?

This would include all treatments, in the judgement of the doctor, which would result in prolonging the dying process. These treatments could include use of a respirator, cardio- pulmonary resuscitation, and maintenance of blood pressure or stable heart rate with medication, transfusion, dialysis, intravenous feedings or feedings via a tube in the stomach. Means to lessen pain and keep you comfortable would be continued.

WHO DETERMINES WHEN I AM NO LONGER ABLE TO MAKE MY OWN MEDICAL DECISIONS?

Your physician determines when you are no longer capable of making your own health care decisions.

HOW IS A DURABLE POWER OF ATTORNEY DIFFERENT THAN A LIVING WILL?

In this document, you name another person as your health care agent, an individual who will make medical decisions for you if you are no longer capable. You can also include specific instructions on possible treatments

IS IT IMPORTANT TO HAVE BOTH A LIVING WILL AND A DURABLE POWER OF ATTORNEY?

The living will takes effect when there is no hope for recovery, while the durable power of attorney is necessary when you are unable to make medical decisions, which may be a temporary state. It is therefore worthwhile to have both documents.

CAN THE INDIVIDUAL I NAME AS A DURABLE POWER OF ATTORNEY HANDLE MY FINANCIAL MATTERS AS WELL?

The durable power of attorney only allows your health care agent to make medical decisions for you. Other decision making issues, such as financial matters can be handled with a different document, a general durable power of attorney.

WHAT ABOUT THE POSSIBILITY OF REVISING OR REVOKING MY ADVANCED DIRECTIVES?

You can cancel or change your directives at any time. You may wish to review your directives periodically or with any major change in your life or medical condition. If you become divorced, your durable power of attorney will be revoked if your prior spouse was named as your health care agent and an alternate was not named.

WHO SHOULD KEEP COPIES OF MY ADVANCE DIRECTIVES?

Keep the original documents with your other important papers. Your physician, family, and the health care agent named in your durable power of attorney should keep copies. When you are admitted to the hospital, you should bring a copy, which will be placed in the hospital chart.

DO I NEED AN ATTORNEY TO PROVIDE THESE FORMS?

An attorney is not required to create an advanced directive. These forms are readily available at your hospital. Another source is the internet. If you have questions, your physician or staff at the hospital should be able to assist you.

ANY ADDITIONAL RESOURCES FOR ADVANCE CARE PLANNING?

Here are a few:

Project GRACE (www.projectgrace.org). You will find planning tools and a newly revised advance care document, a helpful guide, plus additional resources.

The Medical Directive (www.medicaldirective.org). Here you can download a scenario based living will.

CHAPTER SIXTEEN
HOSPICE CARE AND END OF LIFE

Philosophically, death is a natural passage, an end to life. Death is as natural an occurrence as birth. Without death there would be no room for renewal. It is death which makes our finite lives so precious. It motivates us to grow and develop our capacities, to explore our world and live fully. And yet, in our culture, death is taboo. It is hidden and rarely discussed. Death in modern times rarely occurs at home, but is relegated to the confines of the hospital.

Fear of the unknown and the ultimate unknown, death, is profound. In death we must face the ultimate loss, everything we have held most dear in this life. Many physicians and nurses are uncomfortable dealing with the dying. In death, they see defeat. The potentially curable has not been cured. They may shy away from the dying as their own anxieties on the issue are uncovered. Just as we should aim to live the "good life," we should strive to have a "good death."

Death for some may come rapidly and incomprehensibly after an accident or massive heart attack or stroke or even during sleep. For those with cancer, death often comes slowly as the cancer weakens and destroys the body.

People facing their slow demise go through stages dealing with their death, documented by Elizabeth Kubler Ross in her book, *On Death and Dying*. For most individuals denial is the first coping mechanism (it can't be, I'll recover). After denial, anger often follows. For many, negotiation is part of coping (if I do this and that, maybe I'll get better). In the last stages, in a "good death" comes acceptance. Acceptance of the inevitable and a release of worry, pain, and fear, an appreciation of a life well lived, and time for forgiveness and to say good-bye to your loved ones, all encompass a good death.

The Hospice movement, first started in Europe and now widespread in our country aims to provide each individual with a good death. Trained, compassionate nurses and professionals see to the emotional and physical care of the dying. Dignity is preserved. The family becomes an integral part of the process. The individual passes from this world surrounded by all the care, love and comfort that can be provided. Hospice services are now widely available and can be provided at home, in a hospital, or in a hospice center. Tapping hospice services is appropriate for many individuals facing the final stages of dying with cancer. The daily issues can be overwhelming, even in the most supportive family environment.

For those affiliated with a religious group, clergy can bring additional emotional support. Reinforcing the individual's faith may ease growing fears. Your primary care physician, urologist, oncologist, or hospital social worker can serve as valuable resources in procuring the physical, emotional, and spiritual support you may need in this most difficult time.

GLOSSARY

In the following, you will find helpful terms used in this book. These words are also found in other medical literature and are commonly used by medical professionals.

Abdomen: lower part of the torso between the rib cage and the pelvic bone, containing many internal organs.

Abscess: a collection of pus within the body

Adjuvant therapy: therapy after surgery, usually indicating chemotherapy and or radiation

Adverse reaction: an ill effect from medication or chemotherapy

Anesthesia: generally use of a medication to block pain

Anterior: toward the front

Antibiotic: medication used to kill bacteria

Atelectasis: collapse of lung tissue which may occur after surgery

Autologous transfusion: using an individual's own blood during or after planned surgery

Bacteria: one celled living organisms that can cause infection

BCG: Bacillus Calmette Guerin, a vaccine made from deactivated Tuberculosis bacterium, used to treat bladder cancer

Benign: a non cancerous tumor

Bladder: a muscular organ which stores and expels urine

Bladder neck: a thick muscular ring which encircles the exit part of the bladder through which urine passes

Bladder perforation: an accidental hole made in the bladder during surgery

Bladder spasms: painful contractions of the bladder usually resulting from catheterization, surgery, or irritation

Bilateral: both sides

Biopsy: removal of a small piece of tissue for examination to determine if cancer is present

Blood clot: a solid form of blood

Bone Scan: a nuclear medicine scan of the skeletal system used to detect metastatic spread of cancer to the bones

Bowel prep: cleansing of the bowel and taking antibiotics in preparation for examination or surgery

Cancer: a tumor which can spread beyond its site of origin causing destruction of normal tissue and possibly death

Catheter: a hollow tube used to drain or instill fluids into the body

Catheterize: passing a catheter into a body part

Cell: the smallest unit of the body, cells working together make tissues

Carcinogens: agents which can induce the growth of a cancer

Carcinoma in situ: cancer growing in the mucosal layer

Chemotherapy: the use of medication to kill or suppress cancer

Clinical trial: experimental study using patients to determine if therapy is safe and or effective

Complication: an undesirable result of treatment

Continence: the ability to control the flow of urine from the bladder

Continent diversion: use of bowel to create a pouch which stores urine and requires catheterization to drain

Corpora cavernosa: twin vascular conduits in the penis which can fill with blood resulting in an erection

Computerized Axial Tomography (CT) scan: a computerized composite of X ray images used to create a cross section image of the body

Cytology: microscopic examination of cells to detect cancer

Cystoscope: a fiber optic instrument used to examine the bladder and urethra

Cystoscopy: examination of the bladder accomplished with a scope

Depth of penetration: how deeply a tumor grows into the wall of an organ

Diagnosis: defining a medical condition

Dissection: surgical removal of tissue

DNA: Deoxyribonucleic acids are molecules in the cell which carry the information for normal cell function

Differentiation: the degree of specialization of a cell which is lost to various degrees when cancer develops

Enterostomy nurse: an individual trained to care for and instruct individuals with ostomies

Epidural: the space just outside the spinal canal where a small line can be placed temporarily for injections of anesthetics for pain control

Erectile dysfunction: inability to maintain an erection adequate for sexual relations

Frozen section: rapid microscopic analysis by a pathologist, accomplished by freezing a biopsy, during surgery

General anesthesia: a state of unconsciousness achieved through medication to allow surgery to be done without sensation or awareness

Grade: an assessment of the loss of differentiation of a cell when cancer develops, a higher grade would indicate less differentiated and potentially more serious cancer

Gross Hematuria: visible blood in the urine

Hematuria: blood in the urine

High grade: poorly differentiated cancer which is aggressive and more likely to spread and be deadly

ICU: intensive care unit, a specialized area of the hospital where critically ill patients can be managed and treated most effectively

Ileal loop: a form of urinary diversion using a piece of ileum

Ileum: a section of small bowel

Ileus: delayed return of bowel function resulting in abdominal distention

Immune system: the body's cellular defense system which fights infection and cancer

Immunotherapy: therapy based on triggering or enhancing the body's immune response, or providing cells or components of the immune response to fight cancer or disease

Interferon: immunotherapy to fight cancer

Intravesical therapy: therapy placed into the bladder to prevent or treat cancer

Intravenous: into the vein, such as inserting an intravenous line to infuse fluid or medication

Intravenous pyelogram: an X ray image of the kidneys, ureters, and bladder, utilizing intravenous contrast

Invasive bladder cancer: a bladder cancer that grows beyond the mucosal lining layer into the lamina propria or deeper into the muscle

"-itis": suffix which appears after many medical terms, indicating infection or inflammation of that tissue, as in cystitis (infection or inflammation of the bladder)

IV: intravenous (into or through the vein)

Kidney: paired organs located in the abdomen which make urine

Lamina propria: the layer of cells and blood vessels between the superficial mucosa of the bladder and the deeper muscle layers

Local anesthesia: use of anesthesia to create numbness in a part of the body

Local plus sedation: use of local anesthesia plus intravenous sedation

Local recurrence: return of cancer to its original site of origin

Lymph: fluid which bathes the cells of the body, carrying cells to fight infection and cancer

Lymphatic system: a network of channels and nodes which carry lymph throughout the body

Lymph node: small bean shaped structures located throughout the body that filter lymph

Lymph node dissection: removal of lymph nodes around an organ usually accomplished during surgery for cancer

Malignant tumor: a cancerous tumor which is potentially deadly

Metastatic tumor: a cancer which has spread beyond the normal confines of the organ of origin via lymphatics or veins

Microscopic: too small to see with the eye, seen only with a microscope

Microscopic hematuria: blood in the urine visible only under the microscope

Moderately differentiated: intermediate grade cancer

MRI: magnetic resonance imaging, a machine which uses magnets to create images of the body

Multi-focal: multiple foci or sites, usually referring to multiple tumors

Muscularis mucosa: the few muscle fibers located in the superficial stromal layer of the bladder called the lamina propria

Muscularis propria: the thick muscle layer of the bladder

Mutation: an alteration in the genetic makeup of the cell which can result in the growth of a cancer

Negative biopsy: a biopsy which fails to show a specific disease or cancer

NG tube: nasogastric tube, a tube inserted through the nose into the stomach

Neobladder: a urinary diversion in which bowel is attached to the urethra

Neoadjuvant: chemotherapy or radiation given prior to surgery

Organ: tissues working together for a specific function, such as the bladder

Oncologist: a medical specialist trained in the delivery of chemotherapy

Ostomy: a diversion of the bowels or urinary tract; ileostomy, colostomy, urostomy

Papillary tumor: delicate, frond like tumor usually superficial and low grade

Pathologist: a physician who is a specialist in examining tissue and microscopic specimens to determine if disease or cancer is present

Permanent section: final analysis of tissue by a pathologist after proper staining and fixation of the specimen

Pneumonitis: inflammation or infection of the lung

Poorly differentiated: a high grade aggressive cancer with a poor prognosis

Positron Emission Tomography (PET) scan: a device which uses positron emitting radioisotopes to create a computerized image which can be used to detect cancer

Positive biopsy: a biopsy showing cancer

Positive margin: cancer found at the cut end of tissue removed from the body indicating the possibility that some cancer may remain behind

Posterior: toward the back

Pre-op: prior to surgery

Primary Care Physician: a physician who manages the overall care of an individual, often involved in the coordination of specialists

Prognosis: predicting outcome or long term chance of recovery

Progression: cancer which returns in a more serious form

Pulmonary embolus: a blood clot which forms in the veins and travels up into the lungs

Radiation oncologist: a specialist who treats cancer patients with radiation therapy

Recovery room: the specialized area where patients recover after surgery prior to being sent home or to their hospital rooms

Renal pelvis: the main drainage area of each kidney

Resectoscope: a special scope used to cut away tissue in the bladder and urethra

Recurrence: return of cancer

Sepsis: an illness which results in the release of toxins, leading to a breakdown of bodily functions often leading to death

Sessile tumor: solid appearing tumor usually high grade and invasive

Sign: a physical finding related to an abnormality or disease

Spinal anesthesia: anesthesia resulting from injecting the spinal cord with medication to temporarily block pain

Symptom: an individual's feeling or experience caused by a disease

Stage: a system which describes the size, penetration, and degree of spread of a cancer

Stoma: the end of the ostomy which protrudes through the skin

Superficial bladder cancer: a bladder cancer confined to the lining layer or mucosa

Tertiary Care Hospital: usually a teaching hospital that often provides a high level of specialty services

Transitional cells: cells comprising the inner lining or urothelium of the kidneys, ureters, bladder and part of the urethra

Transitional cell cancer: the most common cancer developing anywhere in the urothelium of the urinary tract.

Transurethral resection: removal of a tumor with a special scope which is passed through the urethra

Toxicity: serious side effects of chemotherapy agents

Tumor: abnormal tissue growth either benign or malignant

Ureter: the muscular conduit which carries urine from each kidney to the bladder

Urethra: the muscular conduit which carries urine from the bladder to outside the body

Urethrectomy: removal of the urethra

Urologist: a doctor who specializes in diseases of the male and female urinary tracts and the male reproductive system

Urostomy: a reconstruction of the urinary tract

Urothelium: the lining layer of cells throughout the urinary system, involving the kidneys, ureters, bladder, and urethra

Vesical: medical term for bladder

APPENDIX

ADDITIONAL SOURCES FOR INFORMATION

The following appendix lists additional sources which may provide valuable information and insight into the treatment of bladder cancer. These organizations can also provide the individual and the family with help in coping with the illness.

American Association for Cancer Research
www.aacr.org

American Cancer Society
Local office for the Society will be listed in the white pages of your phone book.
www.cancer.org
by phone: 800-227-2345
by mail: 1599 Clifton Road NE
        Atlanta, GA 30329-4251

American Foundation for Urologic Disease
www.afud.org
by phone: 800-242-2383
by mail: AFUD
        1000 Corporate Boulevard
        Suite 410
        Linthicum, MD 21090

American Society of Clinical Oncology
www.asco.org
by phone: 703-299-0150
by mail: 1900 Duke Street, Suite 200
Alexandria, VA 22314

Cancer Information Service of the National Cancer Institute
www.nci.nih.gov/cancer-information/cancer type/bladder/
by phone: 800-422-6237
by mail: Office of Cancer Communications
National Cancer Institute
Building 31, Room 10A16
Bethesda, MD 2089

International Cancer Alliance (ICARE)
www.icare.org
by phone: 800-ICARE-61 or 301-654-7933
by mail: 4853 Cordell Avenue, Suite 11
Bethesda, MD 20814

National Cancer Institute
www.nci.nih.gov
by phone: 800-422-6237
by mail: National Cancer Institute Public Information Office
Building 31, Room 10A31
31 Center Drive, MSC 2580
Bethesda, Maryland 20892-2580

National Coalition for Cancer Survivorship
www.cansearch.org/
by phone: 301-650-8868
by mail: National Coalition for Cancer Survivorship
1010 Wayne Ave, 5th Floor
Silver Springs, MD 20910

National Center for Complementary and Alternative Medicine
nccam.nih.gov
by phone: 1-888-644-6226
by mail: NCCAM Clearinghouse, P.O. Box 7923
                Gaithersburg, Maryland 20898

National Comprehensive Cancer Network
www.nccn.org
by phone: 888-909-6226
by mail: National Comprehensive Cancer Network
                50 Huntingdon Pike, Suite 200
                Rockledge, PA 19046

INDEX

D

Death 102, 122
Delerium tremens 71
Depression 116
Depth of penetration 20, 42, 43, 44, 126
Diagnosis 27, 28, 29, 30, 31, 32, 33, 126
Diet, relation to bladder cancer 115
Diverticuli 52
Dome, bladder 52, 53, 65, 69
Doxorubicin 64
Drain 79, 80, 81, 125
Durable power of attorney 118, 119, 120

E

Endotracheal tube 48, 72, 76
End of life care 118
Enterostomy nurse 72, 126
Erectile dysfunction 79, 105, 126
  Causes 106
  Definition 105
  Mechanics of erection 106
  Nerve sparing surgery 106, 107
  Radical cystcclomy, association with 80
  Treatment 108
Experimental therapy 101
Extracoporeal shock wave Lithotripsy (ESWL) 86

F

Female sexual dysfunction 80
Fleets phosphosoda 71
Food and Drug Administration (FDA) 111

G

General anesthesia 48, 126
Grade, bladder cancer 20, 21, 22
  Description 126
  Likelihood of spread 19, 20

Gross hematuria 24
Guided imagery 72, 114

H

Health care agent 119, 120
Hematuria
  Causes 24, 25
  Work up 25
Herbal remedies 70, 112
High grade, bladder cancer 20, 29, 40, 43, 44, 56, 57, 58, 59, 68, 129
  Prognosis 20, 30, 34, 39, 43, 44, 45, 57, 68, 129
  Stage 34
Hospice care 122
Hydroureteronephrosis 56

I

Ileus 80, 126
Immune system 126
Immunotherapy 63, 127
Incontinence 91, 93
Inferior vena cava 82
Initial evaluation for bladder cancer 23
Intensive care unit 77, 126
Interferon 63, 64, 127
  Combination with BCG 64
  Effectiveness 64
  Side effects 64
Intracavemosal injection 108
Intravenous line 47, 72, 73, 78, 100, 127
Intravenous pyclogram (IVP) 31
Intravesical therapy 59
  Candidates for 59
  Chemotherapy 59, 64, 65
    Drugs 64
    Effectiveness 65
Invasive, bladder cancer 67
  Cure 68
  Grade 69
  Initial treatment 69
  Partial cystectomy 69

Printed in the United States
63514LVS00004B/213

9 781420 863659